CW00322526

Spongiform Encephalopathy Advisory Committee

Transmissible Spongiform Encephalopathies

A Summary of Present Knowledge and Research

September 1994

London: HMSO

15. MY 1995

464196

		Page
Summary		7
SEAC Membership		8
Preface		9
Introduction		10

Chapter 1   An Introduction to Transmissible Spongiform Encephalopathies

1.1	Preamble	11
1.2	Historical perspective	11
1.3	Slow infections	12
1.4	Experimental scrapie	13
1.5	Inactivation of scrapie-like agents	13
1.6	Pathogenesis of experimental scrapie in mice	14
1.7	Scrapie strains, cloning and mutation	15
1.8	Genetics - The *PrP* gene in sheep and in man - general considerations	17
1.9	The role of the *Sinc* gene in mice	17
1.10	Transgenic mice, TSEs and cell culture	18
1.11	Deletion of the *PrP* gene	18
1.12	The species barrier	18
1.13	*Pr*ion *P*rotein or *P*rotease *r*esistant *P*rotein (PrP)	19
1.14	Differentiation of normal and abnormal forms of PrP	20
1.15	PrP and strains of agent	20
1.16	Pathology	20
1.17	Non-transmissible spongiform encephalopathies	20
1.18	*Post mortem* confirmation of scrapie-like diseases including detection of PrP	21
1.19	The causal agent of TSEs	23
1.20	Explanations for the existence of agent strains	24
1.21	Development of *in vivo* tests for infectivity to assist disease control	24
1.22	Disease prevention by chemotherapy	24
1.23	Infection, contagion and experimental transmission	24
1.24	The incidence, epidemiology and clinical features of TSEs	25
	– Human TSEs	25
	– Kuru	25
	– Creutzfeldt-Jakob disease (CJD)	25
	– Gerstmann-Sträussler-Scheinker syndrome (GSS)	26
	– *PrP* gene mutations in CJD, GSS and Fatal Familial Insomnia (FFI)	26
	– Animal TSEs	27
	– Scrapie in sheep	27
	– Scrapie in goats	27
	– BSE	27
	– SE in captive wild ruminants, domestic cats and captive wild FELIDAE	28
	– Chronic wasting disease (CWD)	29
	– Transmissible mink encephalopathy (TME)	29
1.25	Summary and conclusions	29
	Reading list	30

Chapter 2 Epidemiology

2.1	Scrapie history and epidemiology	33
2.2	Bovine spongiform encephalopathy	35
	– Control	36
	– Maternal transmission	38
	– Effects of the ruminant protein ban of 18 July 1988	39
	– BSE in animals born after July 1988	40
	– Changes in the epidemic	42
	– BSE in other countries	43
	– Suspect BSE cases that are negative for BSE	44
2.3	New SEs of other species	44
2.4	The effectiveness of commercial rendering on the inactivation of scrapie and BSE agents	45
2.5	Human transmissible spongiform encephalopathy	46
	Reading list	46

Chapter 3 Genetics

3.1	Introduction	49
3.2	Molecular genetics	49
	– Familial disease	49
	– Human genetics	49
	– Genetic variation	51
	– Sheep genetics	51
	– Interaction of *Sip* and agent strain groups in sheep	51
	– Cattle genetics	52
	– *PrP* gene in captive wild ruminants and other species	52
3.3	Population genetics	52
	Reading list	53

Chapter 4 Pathogenesis and Pathology

4.1	Tissue assays and titrations	55
4.2	*Sinc* gene	55
4.3	Pathogenesis of natural scrapie	56
4.4	Pathogenesis in experimental BSE and natural TME	56
4.5	PrP^{Sc} accumulation and cellular changes	57
4.6	Neurohistopathology and PrP^{Sc} detection	58
4.7	Strain typing	59
4.8	Pathogenesis of CNS disease	59
	Reading list	60

Chapter 5 **Transmission**

5.1	Introduction	61
5.2	Agent strains	61
5.3	Efficiency of different routes of infection	62
5.4	Effective exposure	62
5.5	The species barrier	62
5.6	Donor species effect	62
5.7	Natural host range of TSE agents	63
5.8	Transmission from man to man	63
	– Kuru	63
	– Iatrogenic CJD	63
5.9	Transmission from animals to animals	63
	– Iatrogenic scrapie	63
	– Animal TSEs associated with feed	63
5.10	Experimental host range for TSE agents	63
5.11	Tissue assays in sheep with scrapie	64
5.12	Tissue assays in clinical cases of BSE and brain titrations in BSE and scrapie	64
5.13	Pathogenesis, attack rate and concurrent assays/titrations in mice and cattle	64
5.14	Other studies	67
5.15	Transmission from human tissues	67
5.16	Maternal transmission	67
5.17	Embryo transfer (ET) in sheep	67
5.18	Embryo transfer in cattle	68
5.19	Rendering study	69
5.20	Agent inactivation	70
5.21	Risk assessment, CJD surveillance and monitoring	71
	Reading list	72

Chapter 6 **Molecular Studies**

6.1	Introduction	75
6.2	Partially protease resistant protein (PrP)	75
6.3	Tissue culture	77
6.4	Transgenics	77
6.5	Gene sequencing	77
6.6	The nature of the agents of TSEs	78
6.7	Protein only hypothesis	79
6.8	Nucleic acid	80
6.9	Biochemical alterations in scrapie-like diseases	81
	Reading list	81

Addendum to Chapter 6   Some Alternative Hypotheses on the Aetiology of Transmissible Spongiform Encephalopathies

6.10	Introduction	83
	– Intestinal fluid dependent organisms (IFDO)	83
	– Nucleation and crystallisation	83
	– Molecular chaperones	83
	– ssDNA	84
	– Green cluster nutrients and BSE	84
	– Use of high nitrogen fertilisers and BSE	84
	– Organophosphorus compounds (OPC)	84
	– A bacterial hypothesis	84
	– Neuronal cell membrane hypothesis	84
6.11	Comments on alternative hypotheses	85
	Reading list	85

Chapter 7   Recent Research and Some Specific Questions

7.1	Introduction	87
7.2	Recent research	87
7.3	Some specific questions	89
	– The nature of the agent(s)	89
	– The pathological changes	89
	– Transmission	89
	– Control of BSE epidemic	90
	– Important applied questions	90
7.4	Research programmes	90
7.5	**Concluding Remarks** - some implications for research	90
	Reading list	91

Acknowledgements	93
Glossary of Abbreviations and Scientific Terms	95

Summary

This report has been written to explain spongiform encephalopathies (SEs) to a wide variety of people, ranging from administrators to research scientists.

Chapter 1 gives a condensed account of SEs for the general reader but could well be read with profit by general biologists and clinicians and as background for anyone wishing to focus on the later more detailed sections.

The later sections go into more detail. Chapter 2 reviews the epidemiology of SEs of animals and man, with particular attention to that of BSE and includes recent data. Chapter 3 briefly surveys the patchy knowledge we have of the 'conventional' genetics of disease susceptibility and the rapidly expanding results of studies of PrP genetics and disease of animals and man.

Chapter 4 summarises how infectivity develops and travels in the host and the characteristic morphological changes. This leads on to Chapter 5 on transmission which describes some science which is very relevant to the causation and control of disease, including experiments in laboratory animals on the effectiveness of different routes of infection and clinical experience of transmission between human beings. In addition there are comments on studies in progress on important unanswered questions regarding the transmission of BSE and the control of the epidemic.

Chapter 6 surveys the rapidly increasing body of molecular studies particularly on PrP, its nature, structure and metabolism, much of it obtained using exciting new techniques such as transgenic animals and PrP-producing tissue cultures. We conclude however that the question of the basic nature of the agent is still not answered although the riddle might be solved at any time.

The final section indicates where we believe our present knowledge fails, and is set out as unanswered questions of both a general and specific type. Communicating such questions will, we hope, stimulate the initiation of more research, though obviously different research groups will wish or be able to tackle different sets of questions.

This report has had to serve so many purposes that we must crave the indulgence of the many who will find it does not exactly fit their wishes and needs. While making it understandable to some non-scientists we know we have not been able to explain all those terms and concepts which we need to use but which are not common knowledge. On the other hand to avoid congesting the text with detailed references to all statements we have appended to each chapter full references to authoritative reviews and some specific research so that the scientist with a specific point in mind will need to take a moment to go through the authors and titles to find what he or she wants.

This has the strengths and weaknesses of many committee reports. It was assembled from many different contributions and opinions and passed through a series of revisions of both substance and style, but it has the agreement and approval of all the members with their varying experience and expertise. It does not include the very latest results, though after due deliberation we decided to include the results of some research still in progress. Nevertheless, we send it out as a contribution to the open and informed discussion which is regarded as the civilised way to advance science and policy these days, but which demands that participants show a degree of understanding and mature judgement which does not come easily.

Spongiform Encephalopathy Advisory Committee (SEAC) Members

Membership

Dr D A J TYRRELL FRS (CHAIRMAN) - Retired Physician and Virologist

Dr R G WILL (DEPUTY CHAIRMAN) - Consultant Neurologist

PROFESSOR I V ALLEN - Medical Neuropathologist

PROFESSOR F BROWN FRS - Virologist

Dr W D HUESTON (From December 1993) - Veterinary Epidemiologist

Dr R H KIMBERLIN - Consultant on transmissible spongiform encephalopathies

Mr D B PEPPER - Veterinary Surgeon

Dr W A WATSON - Retired Director of the Central Veterinary Laboratory

Professor R M Barlow (Retired in December 1992) - Veterinary Pathologist

Observers

DoH

Dr J HILTON (From: September 1994)
Dr M McGovern (To: August 1994)
Dr A Wight (To: April 1994)
Dr H Pickles (To: September 1991)

MAFF

Mr R BRADLEY

AFRC Permanent Contact

Dr J N Wingfield (To: May 1994)

BBSRC Permanent Contact

Mr B HARRIS (From: May 1994)

MRC Temporary Contact

Dr M JEPSON (From: August 1994)
Dr P Dukes (To: August 1994)
Dr K Levy (To: September 1992)

Secretariat

MAFF

Mr T E D EDDY (From: June 1993)
Mr R C McIvor (To: June 1993)
Mr R C Lowson (To: April 1993)

DoH

Mr C LISTER (From: January 1993)
Mr T Murray (To: January 1993)

Preface

The discovery of bovine spongiform encephalopathy (BSE) in November 1986 rekindled a waning interest in research into the transmissible spongiform encephalopathies of man and animals. In May 1988 a Working Party was established to examine the implications of BSE in relation to both animal health and any possible human health hazards and to advise the Government on any necessary measures. This Working Party on BSE, chaired by Sir Richard Southwood FRS, produced some interim recommendations during 1988 and reported finally in February 1989 (The Southwood Report). In February 1989 a Consultative Committee on Research (CCR) into spongiform encephalopathies (SEs) was formed by the Ministry of Agriculture, Fisheries and Food (MAFF) as a result of a recommendation by Professor Southwood's Working Party. Its remit was to advise the MAFF and the Department of Health (DoH) on research on SEs, including the work in progress or proposed, additional research required and the priorities. An interim report (The Tyrrell Report) concentrating on BSE was prepared in June 1989 and subsequently published.

In April 1990 the CCR was re-established as the Spongiform Encephalopathy Advisory Committee (SEAC) with a wider remit to advise the MAFF and the DoH on matters related to the SEs and effectively assuming the role of the Southwood Working Party and the CCR. A second interim report published in April 1992, this time prepared by the SEAC, indicated that the funding agencies and the scientific community had responded to the first report by launching a substantial number of new research projects.

We believe the time has come to set out our understanding of these diseases since this forms the scientific basis of the advice we give. The objective of this third report is therefore to summarise, in accessible language, what is now known about the transmissible spongiform encephalopathies (TSEs). We aim this report at those who wish to be informed of the current status of research into the TSEs, the questions that recent results have answered, those that are outstanding and those which now require investigation. We do not make recommendations or comment on policy; these are not appropriate to the Committee.

We are indebted to a number of scientists who have reviewed or revised particular chapters of the report; however the views expressed here are the responsibility of the Committee.

Reading list

CONSULTATIVE COMMITTEE ON RESEARCH INTO SPONGIFORM ENCEPHALOPATHIES. INTERIM REPORT (The Tyrrell Report).(1989) MAFF, DoH, London, pp 20.

REPORT OF THE WORKING PARTY ON BOVINE SPONGIFORM ENCEPHALOPATHY. (The Southwood Report).(1989) DoH, MAFF London, pp 35.

SPONGIFORM ENCEPHALOPATHY ADVISORY COMMITTEE. INTERIM REPORT ON RESEARCH. (April 1992) DoH, MAFF, HMSO, London, pp 43.

Introduction

The report covers similar subject areas to those in the first interim report but these have been subdivided within the chapters to enable the reader to focus on the particular subject area of interest. It summarises work done in the United Kingdom (UK) and worldwide. References are mainly restricted to authoritative papers and reviews which are listed at the end of each chapter and can be consulted by those who wish to learn more detail.

We wish the text to be understood by as wide an audience as possible and therefore have kept the technical details to a minimum.

Nevertheless it will be helpful for readers to have some basic knowledge of the TSEs. Chapter 1 has been prepared to fulfil this need.

It serves as an introduction to the field and to subjects such as neuropathology and molecular genetics which may be unfamiliar to the general reader but are essential to the understanding of this group of diseases.

Later chapters deal in more detail and depth with other aspects of the field concluding with a series of research questions. Finally there is a glossary of scientific definitions and acronyms.

An Introduction to Transmissible Spongiform Encephalopathies

1.1 *Preamble*

This chapter deals with a group of diseases, the transmissible spongiform encephalopathies (TSEs), that occur in several species of mammals and are listed in Tables 1.1 and 1.2.

1.2 *Historical perspective*

Scrapie of sheep is a fatal neurological disease known for over 250 years in western Europe where from time to time epidemics have occurred. Always recognised to occur predominantly in certain genetically-related sheep, it is only in recent times that the respective roles of heredity and infection have been elucidated. In the early 1920s the rare human disease we now know as Creutzfeldt-Jakob Disease (CJD) was discovered, followed in 1936 by Gerstmann-Sträussler-Scheinker syndrome (GSS) an even rarer variant which occurred in families with an autosomal dominant form of inheritance (see Glossary). Perhaps the disease that most caught the public attention was kuru, first reported in 1957, and associated with ritual endocannibalism at funerals of tribesmen and women in the Fore-speaking region of the eastern highlands of Papua New Guinea where it was the most common cause of death.

The neuropathology of all these diseases was broadly similar, a spongiform encephalopathy, though each had features that distinguished them

Table 1.1 Naturally occurring transmissible spongiform encephalopathies reported before 1985

Host	Disease		Reported distribution
Man	Kuru		Papua New Guinea Declining to rarity
	Creutzfeldt-Jakob disease (CJD)	– sporadic c. 85% – familial c.<15% – iatrogenic c.1%	Worldwide Rare
	Gerstmann–Sträussler (–Scheinker) syndrome (GSS)	–familial	Worldwide Extremely rare
Sheep Goats	Scrapie		Sheep scrapie – Widely distributed but not reported in Australia, New Zealand and some countries of South America and Europe
Mule deer, Elk	Chronic wasting disease (CWD)		North America Localised
Farmed mink	Transmissible mink encephalopathy (TME)		North America Mainland Europe, rare

from each other. The similarity between the neuropathology of kuru and scrapie was first noted in 1959 in a letter to the Lancet by an American veterinary pathologist, Dr W J Hadlow. By then scrapie had been shown to be experimentally transmissible and so Hadlow recommended that someone should attempt to transmit kuru from human brain to primates. This was done by Gibbs and Gadjusek who successfully transmitted to a chimpanzee. For this and other work with kuru Gadjusek was jointly awarded the Nobel Prize for medicine in 1976.

Diseases in the group comprising scrapie, CJD, GSS and kuru, were described later as the transmissible spongiform encephalopathies. The major criteria at that time for inclusion as a member of the group were:

▲ adult occurrence, long incubation, progressive neurological signs ending in fatality,

▲ experimental transmissibility and

▲ spongiform change in grey matter areas of the brain.

1.3 Slow infections

Although at the time thoughts about virus infections of the nervous system were dominated by acute infections such as poliomyeltis, in 1954 the Icelandic veterinarian Björn Sigurdsson put forward the concept of 'slow infections'. Initially he included several, apparently viral diseases of sheep such as maedi/visna (a complex of respiratory and/or nervous disease) jaagziekte (a transmissible lung cancer) and rida (scrapie) all of which occurred in Iceland and caused serious losses in the Icelandic sheep industry. The common features of these diseases were that they were characterised by:

▲ extremely long incubation periods (usually years)

▲ a chronic and progressive course

▲ lesions restricted usually to one organ system and

▲ a fatal outcome.

Table 1.2 Naturally occurring transmissible spongiform encephalopathies (SE) reported from 1985 onwards. Other than BSE all SEs shown are rare. For number of cases of BSE/FSE/SE see Table 2.2

Host	Disease	First report	Reported distribution
Nyala	SE	1987	England
Cattle	Bovine SE	1987	UK, Republic of Ireland (RoI) Oman, Falkland Is. Switzerland, France, Denmark Portugal, Canada, Germany
Gemsbok +	SE	1988	England
Arabian oryx +	SE	1989	England
Greater kudu	SE	1989	England
Eland +	SE	1989	England
Cat	FSE	1990	British Isles
Moufflon +	Scrapie	1992	England
Puma +	FSE	1992	England
Cheetah +	FSE	1992	Australia*, GB, RoI*
Scimitar - horned oryx +	SE	1993	England

+ Transmission not attempted
*Cheetah presumably exposed in Great Britain (GB) prior to export

Clearly scrapie, CJD and GSS all fitted the criteria to be members of the slow infection group. However, there was no epidemiological, aetiological, clinical or pathological connection between them and the other slow diseases and it soon became clear that 'slowness' was not a property of any one taxonomic group of viruses. Furthermore, the causal agents of the scrapie-like diseases appeared to have unusual properties.

So, scrapie, CJD and GSS were separated again into a group known, at least for a period, as the 'Sub-acute transmissible spongiform encephalopathies caused by unconventional agents'.

▲ Sub-acute refers to the usually slow progression of the disease;

▲ transmissible refers to the ability to experimentally transmit the disease to the same or different species, usually by inoculation;

▲ spongiform refers to the groups of holes (vacuoles) seen in brain tissue sections examined by microscopy;

▲ an encephalopathy is a degenerative condition of the brain;

▲ unconventional refers to the fact that unlike conventional viruses, the agents stimulate no immune response in the host and are extraordinarily resistant to inactivation by ultra-violet and ionising radiation, chemical disinfection and heat; these properties distinguish them from viruses causing other slow diseases;

▲ the term agent was used instead of virus, to indicate this unconventionality and that its nature and structure were unknown.

1.4 *Experimental scrapie*

The first experimental transmissions of natural scrapie were made in France in the late 1930s, first to sheep and then to goats. In the early 1960s mouse, and later hamster, models of experimental scrapie were developed with shorter incubation periods than those in the natural disease, and there was a vast expansion in experimentation.

These studies determined the resistance to physical and chemical treatments: in addition the basic

pathogenesis of experimental scrapie in mice was discovered, including the role of a gene *(Sinc)* that controls the incubation period. The experimental host range and the concept of the species barrier, the characterisation of agent strains and their ability to mutate, were also investigated. The structure of the agent was also studied and methods to detect it in clinical material were sought. This resulted in the identification of the protein PrP and the host gene that produces it. Since many, but not all, isolates of natural scrapie from sheep transmit to mice, the species was used for the assay of scrapie infectivity in sheep tissues, and later for the assay of BSE infectivity in cattle tissues.

1.5 *Inactivation of scrapie-like agents*

The unconventional agents causing TSEs are extraordinarily resistant to physical and chemical treatments that destroy even the most resistant bacteria, spores, fungi and viruses. Wet heat is more destructive to them than dry heat, particularly in the absence of lipids. For example porous load autoclaving at 136-138°C at 30 psi for 18 minutes appears to destroy the most thermostable strains of scrapie agent. Treatment with 1M or 2M sodium hydroxide has inactivated substantially, but not always completely, and sodium hypochlorite solution containing 2 % available chlorine, for 1 hour, is probably the chemical of choice for disinfection. Dichloroisocyanurate (which can yield similar chlorine concentrations to sodium hypochlorite) and formaldehyde are both ineffective decontaminants.

Neither ultraviolet nor ionising radiation have a significant effect except at levels higher than those that could be used with safety in the environment. BSE agent responds like scrapie agent in all these respects. Knowledge of the heat/time/pressure combinations used during commercial rendering that are able to consistently inactivate infected ruminant waste, and thus make the products safe for further use, is of considerable practical importance (see para 5.19).

1.6 *Pathogenesis of experimental scrapie in mice*

In order to study the development of disease from the point of exposure to the onset of clinical signs it is helpful to challenge experimental, susceptible animals in a manner certain to produce the disease, ideally following a short incubation period. This circumvents the difficulties encountered in studying natural disease when it is not known when, or even if, exposure has occurred. Inoculation of mouse-adapted scrapie directly into nervous tissue (brain intracerebral (i/c), spinal cord, peripheral nerve) of mice enables infection to be established directly. If other routes such as sub-cutaneous (s/c), intraperitoneal (i/p) or intravenous (i/v) are used, the infectivity is dispersed widely and rapidly via the blood stream but, as following i/c inoculation, infectivity is eliminated therefrom in a matter of hours. The efficiency of these routes of infection decreases in comparison to the i/c route in the order i/c > i/v > i/p > s/c. The intragastric (alimentary) route has the lowest efficiency requiring about 10^5 (100,000) times more effective LD_{50} units to produce the same effect as a single i/c dose.

Following inoculation and a brief viraemic period there is often a 'zero' phase (Figure 1.1) during which no infectivity can be detected. When peripheral (*ie* non-neural routes) of infection are used, infection of and replication in the spleen and lymph nodes occurs. If the strain of agent and mouse *Sinc* genotype (see para 1.7) permit neuroinvasion, this process is initiated but may not be detected in the brain until approximately half way through the incubation period. Infection reaches the brain from the spleen, probably via the visceral sympathetic fibres of the splanchnic nerve. The splanchnic nerve carries such fibres to and from the spleen to the spinal cord. Infection then enters the spinal cord in the mid thoracic region and passes caudally (towards the tail) and rostrally (towards the head; literally beak) to the brain at a maximum rate of about 1 mm per day. In the brain replication occurs to a higher titre (amount of

Figure 1.1 Scheme of titre changes during incubation of experimental scrapie in mice after parenteral inoculation.

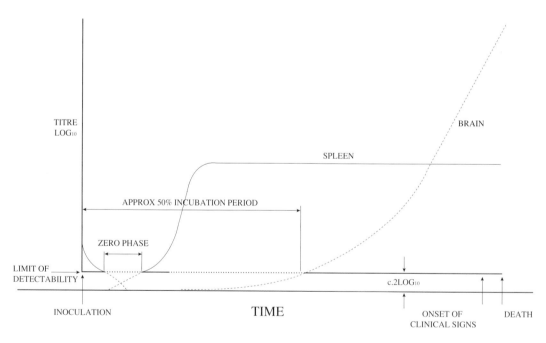

Following parenteral inoculation of mice infectivity quickly declines and becomes undetectable. After an interval (zero phase) infectivity becomes detectable in the spleen, rises as replication occurs and then levels off. Agent can be detected in the nervous system approximately at the mid point of the incubation period and rises rapidly to exceed the titre present in the spleen. The test is only able to detect infectivity at titres of more than 100 infectious doses/g. It should be noted that other models using different mouse and/or scrapie strains may show different time courses and patterns.

Adapted from: Dickinson A G and Outram G W. (1979) The scrapie replication-site hypothesis and its implications for pathogenesis. In: Slow Transmissible Diseases of the Nervous System vol. 2. S B Prusiner and W J Hadlow, eds. Academic Press, New York, pp 13-31.

infectivity) than is maximally reached in the spleen. Once infection has reached the spinal cord and brain it can also pass centrifugally to the peripheral nervous system and this may account for the detection of low and inconsistent infectivity in some peripheral tissues of clinically affected animals.

Splenectomy in the early phase of infection delays neuroinvasion. In the absence of the spleen, infection, replication and neuroinvasion result probably from lymph nodes. After intragastric infection Peyer's patches, which are lymphoid tissue within the gut wall, assume the role of the spleen. This clearly has relevance in natural scrapie and in BSE too where oral (alimentary) infection is the most likely route. In experimental BSE in cattle infectivity has been found in the distal ileum (small intestine closest to the large intestine) in the early stages of incubation (see paras 4.4 and 5.13).

The cells within the lymphoreticular system (LRS) responsible for replication are 'fixed' cells, resistant to radiation; not the mobile cells such as lymphocytes. Follicular dendritic cells may be those in which replication occurs.

For clinical disease to result (which presents with neurological signs) it is necessary for infection and damage to occur in the clinical target areas (CTAs) in the brain. Thus when imprecise inoculations are made directly into the brain much of the brain damage (which may be considerable) is irrelevant to pathogenesis. What is important is that CTAs are infected and functionally disturbed or structurally damaged. This is more readily achieved by precise (stereotactic) inoculation of specific brain sites and by peripheral routes which initially infect the thoracic spinal cord, and thus give more direct access to the CTAs, than via imprecise i/c inoculation.

1.7 *Scrapie strains, cloning and mutation*

Scrapie is a natural disease only of sheep, goats and moufflon (a primitive relative of the sheep). When experimentally transmitted to mice or hamsters it is known as murine (or mouse) scrapie or hamster scrapie respectively. Scrapie does not occur naturally in these species. The first indication of the existence of scrapie strains came from experimental studies in the early 1960s in goats when two clinical

forms of scrapie, 'scratching' and 'drowsy', were determined. Genetic control of the incubation period of experimental scrapie in mice is governed by the *Sinc* gene which has two alleles s^7 (short incubation) and p^7 (prolonged incubation). (*Note* In this publication all genes are italicised, for example *Sinc* gene, *PrP* gene, to distinguish them from their protein products such as PrP which are not italicised). One group of murine scrapie strains, typified by the strain ME7, have short incubations in s^7s^7 mice and much longer incubations in p^7p^7 mice. Another group of strains typified by the strain 22A have the reverse properties. Individual members of each strain group can be distinguished by certain pathological features and, in particular, the lesion profile (that is the distribution within the brain of spongiform change and its severity) and by the length of the incubation period within particular mouse genotypes including F_1 hybrids, that is *Sinc* s^7p^7. In the latter, different strains show different patterns of dominance.

When mixed strains are passaged into a susceptible host genotype the strain with the shortest incubation is always selected and this clearly has a biological advantage for that agent. However, when a 'slow' strain, that is one with a long incubation period, is inoculated in advance of a 'fast' strain, the disease produced is characteristic of the 'slow' strain. This argues for a limited number of replication sites which, once occupied (in this case by the slow strain), permit only the strain first occupying the site to replicate. Individual strains can be isolated from a mixture by cloning, that is by serial passage at limiting dilution into further mice so that the incubation period and lesion profile become stable.

Mutation is a natural phenomenon and is a feature of conventional organisms (viruses and bacteria), and it may result in modification to the virulence of the organisms and clinical signs, pathogenesis and pathology of the disease. Scrapie-like agents are no different in this respect and mutants which are continually being produced will be selected during serial passage within the same host genotype of the species if they confer the biological advantage of a shorter incubation period than that of the parent strain. When cross-species transfers are made experimentally (*eg* mouse scrapie inoculated into rats and hamsters, Figure 1.2) or naturally, as some suggest from sheep with scrapie to cattle, mutant strains may be selected by the new species because they have a biological advantage, and if they have, they may have quite different properties from the parent strain. One of the altered properties may be an increase, or decrease, in pathogenicity of the BSE agent from cattle for other species so the

consequences must be considered and action taken to control the risks if deemed necessary.

It is important to recognise that the strains of agent obtained in mice from isolates from sheep may be selected minor strains, or indeed mutant strains, and so they may not represent the strains occurring in the natural host.

Figure 1.2 The effects on incubation periods of serial passage of mouse scrapie across the species barrier to hamsters and rats

Incubation periods of scrapie strain 139A cloned in the mouse and passed into hamsters and rats

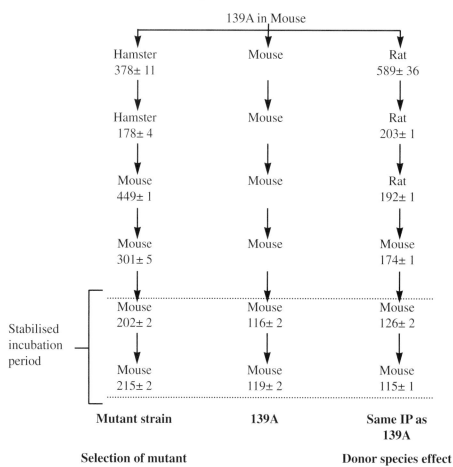

IP = incubation period (days ± SEM)

Different effects of intracerebral passage of cloned strain 139A mouse scrapie through hamsters and rats, followed by re-isolation in *Sinc* s⁷s⁷ mice (to illustrate the DONOR SPECIES EFFECT when there is no change in stable incubation period, and the SELECTION of a MUTANT strain of different stable incubation period).

Adapted from: Kimberlin RH. (1991) Agent-host interactions and pathogenesis. In: Sub-acute Spongiform Encephalopathies. Edited by R Bradley, M Savey and B A Marchant. Current Topics in Veterinary Medicine and Animal Science, vol. 55, pp. 137-147. Kluwer Academic Press, Dordrecht, The Netherlands.

1.8 *Genetics - The PrP gene in sheep and in man - general considerations*

All diseases have a hereditary (genetic) and an environmental component to their aetiology, but the relative importance of these components varies between diseases. Diseases with a strong genetic component are exhibited in families. The TSEs are no exception. For example GSS of man presents as a disease caused by an autosomal dominant gene, which occurs in close relatives according to normal Mendelian laws. However, as with all the TSEs, GSS is experimentally transmissible to primates and some other species by inoculation. At the other end of the spectrum goats appear to be uniformly susceptible to scrapie following experimental challenge and presumably also after natural exposure. Sheep occupy an intermediate position in which a gene *Sip*, controls the length of the incubation period in both the experimental and natural disease, at least in some sheep breeds. *Sip* is probably the ovine equivalent of the murine *Sinc* gene, and PrP^c (see para 1.13) specific to the species may be the gene product of each. The incubation period of scrapie in sheep of some *Sip* genotypes may be so long as to exceed the commercial lifespan of the animals, thus giving a superficial appearance of resistance to disease. This resistance can sometimes be overcome by more challenging, unnatural routes of exposure (such as intracerebral (i/c) inoculation) at high dose.

By challenging sheep with a subcutaneous injection of a standard, pooled inoculum of sheep brain (Sheep Scrapie Brain Pool 1 = SSBP 1) it is possible to generate lines of sheep by conventional breeding methods, which are susceptible or relatively resistant to natural scrapie. This method of identifying sheep is impractical for use on farms, so it was of great importance when a genetic linkage between the *Sip* gene and the *PrP* gene was established in some breeds of sheep. This has made it possible to identify, with reasonable certainty, sheep of some breeds as resistant or susceptible to natural or experimental scrapie, by establishing their genotype with a simple blood test.

This test involves extracting DNA from the white blood cells and sequencing the *PrP* gene, in whole or in part, to detect variations (polymorphisms) in the nucleotide sequences which may code for different amino acids, and thus proteins, which are associated with susceptibility to scrapie. Alternatively DNA can be exposed to selected restriction endonuclease enzymes (which cut DNA at specific sites); different alleles can then be detected by determining the molecular sizes of the cut fragments. (A fuller explanation is given in the Glossary under the heading 'Genes and gene function').

These methods have been employed in a few, mainly experimental flocks, with some success. However, considerable expansion of the work is required because not all breeds appear to have the same genetic markers for susceptibility to scrapie and also it is not known if all naturally occurring scrapie strains interact in the same way with a particular sheep *PrP* genotype. In fact studies of experimental scrapie have shown that sheep which are resistant to one strain of scrapie may be susceptible to a different strain. Clearly if a similar situation occurred with the natural disease it could be risky to breed for 'resistance' to one strain because this could lead to a flock that was susceptible to scrapie of another strain. In cattle, polymorphisms have been found in the *PrP* gene, though there is no apparent association with disease occurrence. In humans with familial forms of TSE, analysis of the *PrP* gene structure is valuable in establishing the responsible pathogenic mutation(s) and may also be used to assess the risk of disease occurrence in unaffected family members. Moreover, the genotype of polymorphic codon 129 of the *PrP* gene appears to influence the phenotype of different pathogenic mutations, as well as susceptibility to sporadic and iatrogenic forms of TSE. One such phenotype is fatal familial insomnia (FFI) (see para 1.24 sub-para "PrP gene mutations in CJD, GSS and FFI and para 2.5).

1.9 *The role of the Sinc gene in mice*

It appears that *Sinc* may control scrapie pathogenesis at two different sites: first at the LRS/neural interface by determining whether the agent can move from an LRS cell to a nerve cell, and second within the nervous system where it controls the rate of replication and/or cell to cell spread. It probably has little influence on the LRS phase of infection. The first control determines whether or not disease is possible since, in some experimental scrapie infections, infectivity develops and persists in the spleen but does not move to the CNS, and there is no disease. If this same agent strain is inoculated into the brain directly, thus bypassing the LRS, scrapie results. It is possible that the *Sip* gene of sheep operates in the same way.

1.10 *Transgenic mice, TSEs and cell culture*

Modern molecular genetic methods enable the genes of mammals to be copied and multiplied in the test tube or in bacteria. Such genes can be modified in many ways. A normal or modified gene can be introduced into embryos from a healthy animal, such as a mouse, so that the effect of the gene can be studied in the progeny of these embryos, and these methods have been used to show the importance of PrP in TSEs. Furthermore, a particular *PrP* gene mutation that is associated with GSS in man has been introduced into mice which have then spontaneously developed a spongiform encephalopathy. It is not yet confirmed whether the induced disease is transmissible, as is its natural counterpart.

Another approach has been to introduce hamster *PrP* genes into mice and then to challenge the mice with either hamster or mouse-adapted scrapie agent. Mice 'transgenic' for the hamster gene and challenged with hamster agent behave precisely like hamsters and unlike mice in this respect. Uninoculated older mice with a high copy number of introduced hamster, sheep or mouse *PrP* genes have also developed a spontaneous and diffuse necrotising myopathy, demyelinating polyneuropathy and focal vacuolation in the central nervous system. In other words the experimental introduction of excessive copies of the *PrP* gene has resulted in the spontaneous development of widespread muscle cell death, loss of fatty myelin 'insulation' from peripheral nerve fibres and microscopic 'holes' within the brain and spinal cord. How and why this has occurred is unknown but is under investigation. These examples of transgenic experiments will no doubt be followed by others and could resolve some of the unknowns about TSEs.

For instance it may be possible to produce transgenic animals highly susceptible to many strains of TSE pathogens, thus making bioassays faster, cheaper and more sensitive. Transgenic cell lines may also be developed and might accomplish the same objectives *in vitro* and so do away with experimental animals altogether for certain purposes. We welcome this approach.

1.11 *Deletion of the PrP gene*

Modern molecular genetic procedures have been employed to delete the *PrP* gene in embryonic mice so that no PrP is produced. This seems to have no apparent effect on growth or the normal development of these so-called 'null' mice to adulthood. They do however have one important new feature. They appear to completely resist development of disease when challenged with scrapie agent to which they would otherwise have been susceptible, and tissues therefrom have no detectable infectivity. Even hemizygous animals (that is mice that have only one copy of the gene instead of the usual two) also show enhanced resistance to scrapie. This shows the importance of PrP and the *PrP* gene in scrapie-like diseases, as will be further discussed in Chapters 3 and 6 of this report.

1.12 *The species barrier*

The transmission of scrapie-like agents is generally more difficult between species than within species, and is most difficult of all by the oral route. Transmission depends on the effective exposure, which comprises the amount of infectivity present in the inoculum, the amount (volume/weight) administered and the route of administration (see paras 5.4 to 5.6). Whether or not disease results is dependent on at least two separate variables - the strain of agent and probably the difference between the *PrP* gene sequence of donor and recipient. If transmission is successful the incubation period is generally longer at the first passage than following a second or third passage. This is called the 'donor species effect' and is perhaps due to the donor PrP^{Sc} functioning less efficiently in the recipient species than the homologous PrP^{Sc} which is generated during the first passage.

1.13 *Prion Protein or Protease resistant Protein (PrP)*

Apart from the microscopic appearance of spongiform change in the brain there is another unique feature of all TSEs. This is the presence, in brain tissue of clinically affected animals, and sometimes in the lymphoreticular tissues (spleen and lymph nodes), of an abnormal form of a host protein called prion protein, or protease resistant protein. This protein is commonly referred to as PrP. It is a sialoglycoprotein *ie* a protein containing sialic acid and carbohydrate groups. The protein is encoded by the *PrP* gene which is widely conserved in mammals. Curiously the function of PrP is unknown despite its presence in many different organs and tissues of healthy animals, including the brain.

Like other proteins PrP is encoded by a specific sequence of nucleotides that constitutes the *PrP* gene. The first process is one of transcription. The genetic message is transmitted by first copying the nucleotide sequence of deoxyribonucleic acid (DNA) to give a messenger ribonucleic acid (mRNA). This process of transcription occurs in the cell nucleus. The mRNA then migrates from the nucleus to the cytoplasm and there directs assembly of amino acids into protein by a process called translation. In this way the *PrP* gene generates the normal cellular form of PrP which is called PrP^C (C = cellular). In the brain, this normal protein is located in the cell membrane of neurons (nerve cells).

In disease the PrP^C is changed to PrP^{Sc} (Sc = scrapie - the generic name for the disease-specific form) (Figure 1.3). The change takes place post-translationally. The nature of the change seems to be conformational, not co-valent *ie* it affects the way the molecule folds but not what chemical bonds are formed; it may form α helix or ß sheet. (These have respectively spiral or pleated, sheet-like shapes, see Darnell *et al* (1990) for a fuller explanation). PrP^C has little or no ß sheet and a high α helix content (42%). By contrast the ß sheet content of PrP^{Sc} is 43% and α helix content 30%. The ß sheet content is even higher (54%) and the α helix content lower (21%) when the protein is treated with Proteinase K (see below and para 1.14) This abnormal folding confers some special properties on the PrP^{Sc} which enable it to be distinguished from its normal counterpart PrP^C, in a number of different ways.

Figure 1.3 Relationships between normal and abnormal PrP forms in central nervous tissues in naturally occurring transmissible spongiform encephalopathies of animals and alternative PrP terminologies

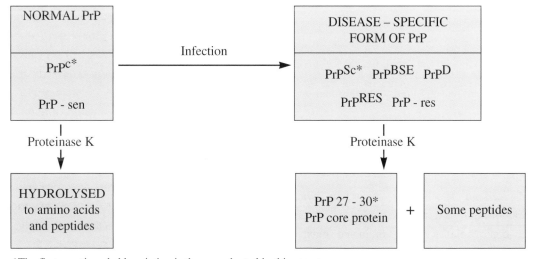

*The first mentioned abbreviation is the one adopted in this report

Infection converts PrP^C to PrP^{Sc}. The two forms of PrP can be distinguished by their response to proteases *eg* Proteinase K. The normal form (PrP^C) is hydrolysed whereas the disease-specific form (PrP^{Sc}) partially resists the treatment and leaves a residue with a lower molecular ratio. Detection of either PrP^{Sc} or PrP 27-30 thus confirms the presence of disease.

Thus in addition to the microscopic spongiform change in brain tissue, it is also possible to detect PrP^{Sc} by immunostaining contiguous tissue sections with antiserum prepared in rabbits against PrP^{Sc}. It is also possible to detect PrP^{Sc} by immunoblotting (Western blotting - see para 1.18). PrP^{Sc} can also be visualised as fibrils, sometimes referred to as scrapie-associated fibrils (SAF) or prion rods, by electron microscopy of detergent extracts of the central nervous system (CNS) of affected individuals. SAFs are resistant to treatment with a proteolytic enzyme, Proteinase K (Figure 1.3).

1.14 *Differentiation of normal and abnormal forms of PrP*

Several different terminologies for the normal and abnormal isoforms of PrP are used in the scientific literature (Figure 1.3). Treatment of unfixed brain (*ie* brain *not* preserved in formalin) with Sarkosyl, a detergent, followed by centrifugation can be used to separate the two PrP isoforms. PrP^{C} is soluble and susceptible to Proteinase K digestion whilst PrP^{Sc} is sedimentable and largely resistant. The insoluble protein resulting from this treatment is called the PrP core protein or PrP27-30 (the figures denote the molecular ratio in kiloDaltons (kDa)). The more commonly used notations for the various forms of PrP, and the relationships between them, are shown in Figure 1.3.

1.15 *PrP and strains of agent*

It has been suggested that variation in the structure of PrP^{Sc} can account for the differences between scrapie strains. PrP^{C} and PrP^{Sc} have a glycosylinositol phospholipid (GPI) terminal which anchors the protein to the cell membrane. Analysis of this anchor in PrP^{Sc} from hamsters has revealed six different glycoforms, of which three are unprecedented. However, identical PrP^{Sc} GPIs were found in two isolates of scrapie (that is different strains of agent) which exhibit different incubation times and lesion profiles. Therefore it does not seem that chemical variation in the structure of the GPI anchor accounts for differences between strains.

Another hypothesis is that different scrapie strains target different populations of neurons which code for cell type-specific PrP. This is unlikely because

agent strain diversity can be demonstrated using inocula prepared from spleen. Furthermore, different agent strains have been propagated in the same tissue culture cell line. However, the simplest and most satisfactory explanation for the existence of strains is the variation in the nucleotide sequence of the assumed nucleic acid genome of the agent. The fact that this has not been discovered is the major failing of the hypothesis to date.

1.16 *Pathology*

Encephalopathy is the term given to describe a degenerative disorder of the brain. An encephalopathy is distinct from an encephalitis, which is an inflammatory process caused, for example, by bacteria or viruses. Encephalitis is usually recognised microscopically by the presence of cellular infiltrations, mostly from the blood and often accompanied in the CNS by a cellular response from resident cells, the microglia and astroglia (supporting cells) and accompanied by the presence of antigen derived from the causal organism. In encephalopathies, inflammatory cells originating from the blood are usually absent, though astroglial reactions and microglial responses are prominent. Spongiform refers to a histological (microscopic) feature in which small round or oval holes (vacuoles) are identified in nerve cell bodies (neuronal perikarya) and their processes (neurites) (Figures 1.4A and 1.4B). Thus these changes are seen predominantly in grey matter (nerve cell rich areas) rather than white matter, which is rich in nerve cell processes (myelinated axons).

1.17 *Non-transmissible spongiform encephalopathies*

There are other encephalopathies which might be confused with TSEs, for example those occurring in liver disease (hepatic encephalopathies). In these the main change is vacuolation of the myelin sheaths of the nerve fibres in the white matter. This contrasts with vacuolation in the nerve cell bodies and their processes in the grey matter in TSEs (Figures 1.4A and 1.4B). The changes in hepatic encephalopathy are due to high blood concentrations of ammonia which result from liver failure, and probably other related metabolic changes. In a proportion of clinically suspect cases of BSE which are not confirmed pathologically, white matter vacuolation has been described and might result from such insults. Although white matter vacuolation may occur in some experimental models of TSEs, it is an inconsistent and usually minor feature in naturally occurring disease.

White tigers between 1970 and 1977, and ostriches between 1986 and 1989, developed neurological illness and brain lesions originally considered to be possible TSEs. However, there is still too little evidence to justify this. Studies are still continuing into the ostrich disease in which the pathological changes are those of an SE.

1.18 *Post mortem confirmation of scrapie-like diseases including detection of PrP*

Suspect TSE cases are usually confirmed *post mortem* by histological examination of areas of the brain where the characteristic features are seen, though the exact areas affected may vary from disease to disease. There may also be loss of neurons (nerve cells) and overgrowth of astroglia, which occurs in many forms of brain damage. Patches or plaques of amyloid protein may also be seen in the extracellular space and in association with blood vessels. These are recognized by special stains, but may be seen in a variety of other diseases of the nervous system. Those that occur in TSEs not only stain positively with conventional histochemical stains for amyloid such as Congo red, but also with antisera to PrP^{Sc} (see para 1.13). Amyloid that occurs in diseases other than TSEs *eg* Alzheimer's disease (AD) can thus be distinguished, because this form of amyloid does not react with sera containing anti-PrP antibodies.

Western blotting or immunoblotting is a method of detecting PrP^{Sc} and can be used to diagnose scrapie-like diseases. In outline, the method consists of

Figure 1.4A Neuronal vacuolation

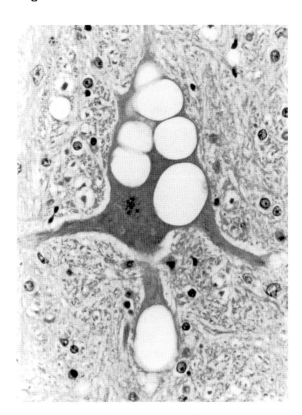

A single nerve cell containing multiple vacuoles.

Figure 1.4B Spongiform change in grey matter neuropil

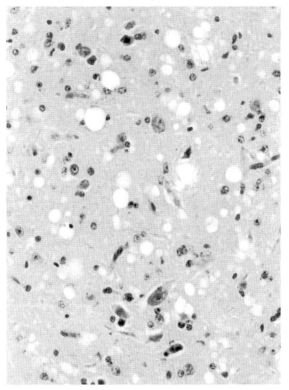

So many nerve cell processes contain vacuoles that the area begins to look like a sponge.

These figures are micrographs of 5μm sections of brain prepared from formalin-fixed tissue embedded in paraffin wax and stained with haematoxylin and eosin.

Figures courtesy of Mr G A H Wells and Mr S A C Hawkins.

21

extracting and purifying the PrP^{Sc} from the CNS, analysing the purified protein by polyacrylamide gel electrophoresis (PAGE), transferring it to a membrane by blotting and then staining this with anti-PrP^{Sc} serum (Figures 1.5A and 1.5B). Thus, at least four methods of laboratory diagnosis of scrapie-like diseases are now available:

Using fixed tissue:

▲ Microscopic examination of stained tissue sections of brain for evidence of spongiform encephalopathy and associated lesions.

▲ Microscopic examination of tissue sections immunostained for PrP^{Sc}.

Using unfixed tissue: (Note: electron microscopy and immunoblotting are effective for detecting fibrils and PrP^{Sc} respectively in autolysed tissue).

▲ Electron microscopy for detection of disease-specific fibrils such as scrapie associated fibrils (SAF) or BSE fibrils (Figure 1.6) in tissue extracts.

▲ Immunoblotting to detect PrP^{Sc}. More sophisticated developments of this method include dot blots using tissue extracts, and histoblots using cryostat (frozen) sections of brain tissue.

However, none of these methods can be regarded as certain and valid means of diagnosis in all circumstances, though singly or collectively they usually permit a confident diagnosis to be reached.

Recent advances have enabled detection of PrP^{Sc} in lymphoreticular tissues of naturally-infected sheep, and of mice experimentally infected with scrapie,

Figure 1.5A
Figure 1.5B

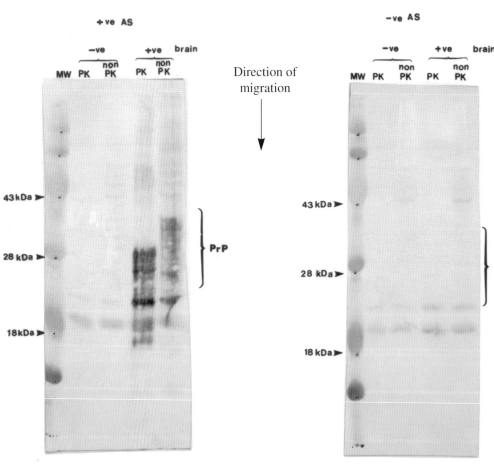

Direction of migration

Extracts of brains from normal and BSE affected cattle have been examined by immunoblotting using A) positive anti-PrP serum and B) negative anti-PrP serum. Figure 1.5A shows PrP in the infected brain which is partly degraded (reduced in molecular mass) by Proteinase K treatment. Bands of molecular mass 19, 22 and 43 kDa are non-specific.

Figures courtesy of Mrs P Keyes.

but the techniques are not yet sufficiently well developed to be employed routinely in non-specialist laboratories. Only microscopic examination of the brain can definitively confirm spongiform encephalopathy and this method also has the advantage that certain alternative or additional diagnoses may be established or eliminated.

1.19 *The causal agent of TSEs*

There are numerous hypotheses for the structure of the causal agent of TSEs. In recent years three main hypotheses have dominated the scene. In one (the prion hypothesis) the agent is defined as a small proteinaceous infectious particle, or prion, that resists inactivation by procedures modifying nucleic acids and that contains PrP^{Sc} as a major and necessary component. This hypothesis does not exclude the presence of a small nucleic acid, but it is not an essential requirement and supporters of the hypothesis are increasingly equivocal about its existence. The way that prions may be propagated is not known but it is suggested that exogenous PrP^{Sc} forms catalytic heterodimers with host PrP^{C}, which results in the formation of more PrP^{Sc}. (In the context of PrP^{Sc} synthesis a heterodimer is an intermediate protein duplex (dimer) consisting of one molecule of PrP^{C} and one of PrP^{Sc} which produces, by an unknown mechanism, two molecules of PrP^{Sc}). There is very little experimental support for this idea but there is a precedent with another protein, p53, in which co-translation of wild type and mutant proteins of differing conformation enforces conversion of the wild type into the mutant form.

Figure 1.6 BSE fibrils

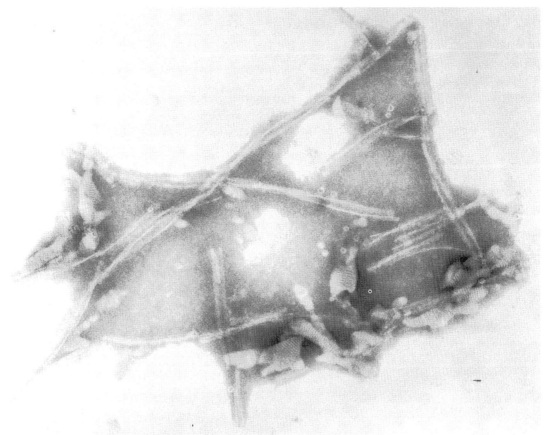

Detergent extracts of unfixed bovine brain from a confirmed case of BSE were treated with Proteinase K, negatively stained and examined by transmission electron microscopy. The unstained fibrils of PrP^{Sc} (indistinguishable from SAF) stand out against the background.

Electron micrograph $\times$ 150,000

Figure courtesy of Mr A C Scott.

By contrast, the virino hypothesis views the agent as an informational hybrid, namely an infectious pathogen containing a small, specific core of non-translated nucleic acid (which may code for no product other than copies of itself) associated with one or more cellular proteins, possibly PrP^{Sc} provided by the host. The key element of this hypothesis is that the agent itself has a nucleic acid genome which confers upon it the ability to replicate itself and encode different strains of agent.

A development of the prion hypothesis that attempts to reconcile the prion and virino theories suggests, again without experimental proof, that a holoprion is composed of an apoprion (= PrP^{Sc}) and a coprion, a recruited host cell episomal nucleic acid. The latter is proposed to modify pathogenicity thus conferring a potential for phenotypic variation on the holoprion.

The third hypothesis suggests the agent is an unconventional virus (that is one that can resist conventional methods of inactivation), which consists of a nucleic acid that codes for a protective protein coat. Though currently less supported than formerly, proponents claim that the hypothesis has not been disproved. Quite recently electron microscopy of SAF extracts of experimental hamster scrapie have revealed structures resembling small virus particles. It is premature to consider that these are the scrapie agent and, as the authors concede, more work needs to be done to determine if they are specific for scrapie-like diseases.

1.20 *Explanations for the existence of agent strains*

There is strong evidence that, as with conventional viruses, TSE agents occur as genetically different 'strains' which can mutate and are identified by their different biological properties, as determined by inoculation into specific inbred mouse strains. Also, GSS (see para 1.24) is hereditary but transmissible. Such phenomena are readily explained by the virino and virus hypotheses in modern molecular biological terms because strain-specific nucleic acids are vital components of the hypotheses. The prion hypothesis does not readily explain these phenomena if no nucleic acid is present. The problem for the virus and virino

hypotheses is that no nucleic acid has yet been found. Research is directed towards testing these hypotheses in various ways.

1.21 *Development of in vivo tests for infectivity to assist disease control*

From a practical point of view the ultimate goal is a specific test that could be applied to detect infected individuals before the onset of clinical signs. This would be very important in enabling eradication of scrapie (which has defied control for centuries) from flocks, regions and countries and for providing evidence that would permit certification of freedom from scrapie for trading in live sheep and sheep products. It could also be important to aid the control of other animal diseases like BSE, though this is not an essential requirement for that purpose, and to detect human carriers of infection so that iatrogenic transmission could be avoided and patients could be identified for preventative treatment, if and when this becomes possible.

1.22 *Disease prevention by chemotherapy*

There are drugs and chemicals that inhibit the accumulation of PrP^{Sc} cells in culture and delay the onset of clinical disease in experimental animals. These include sulphated polyanions, Congo red and amphotericin B. More study should be directed towards the mechanisms by which these substances cause their effects. At present they are only effective if administered with, or before, infection so they cannot be regarded as treatments.

1.23 *Infection, contagion and experimental transmission*

TSEs, by definition, are transmissible and, therefore, infectious. Most are not however contagious, that is transmitted by contact. An important exception is sheep scrapie. Other less well documented exceptions include goat scrapie, chronic wasting disease (CWD) and the TSEs of the greater kudu and eland. Maternal transmission of disease (*ie* transmission from dam to offspring), occurs in sheep and perhaps goats, and is probably the way the disease is maintained in such flocks by 'horizontal' or 'lateral' spread (*ie* spread between other individuals), possibly via infected placenta which is eaten or contaminates pasture or buildings. The mechanism of maintenance of CWD infection in some species of North American deer and elk, and TSE infections in the greater kudu and eland in zoos in England, is not known. Maternal transmission of disease does not occur in any human TSE.

1.24 *The incidence, epidemiology and clinical features of TSEs*

Human TSEs

Kuru, a disease geographically localised to the Fore people of the eastern highlands of Papua New Guinea, was first reported in 1957. Kuru is the native word for shivering and is a fitting description of a major sign of the disease, a fine tremor of the head, trunk and limbs which is associated with the insidious onset of ataxia. The tremor and ataxia progressively worsen and later are accompanied by cerebellar and behavioural signs. The latter take the

form of mood changes and hilarity which have given rise to another description for the disease, 'laughing death'. Dementia, if it occurs at all, is preterminal. The clinical phase usually lasts 6-9 months and begins at age 5-35 years. The incubation period following exposure to and consumption of, kuru-infected human tissues at ritual, funereal cannibalistic feasts is from 5 to over 30 years. Since the late 1950s, when these rituals were outlawed, the disease has declined to a very low incidence but a few cases still occur each year, reflecting an incubation period of 40 years or more. Maternal transmission has not been reported in kuru.

Creutzfeldt-Jakob disease (CJD), first reported in 1920, is a rare disease of worldwide distribution which occurs mainly in the 5th and 6th decades of life with an annual incidence of about 1 case per 2 million. There is no significant association with occupation, place of residence or eating habits. Despite intense epidemiological study there is no evidence that scrapie of sheep is a source of

Figure 1.7 Diagram of the human *PrP* gene open reading frame showing, by codon/amino acid number, mutations and polymorphisms associated with disease

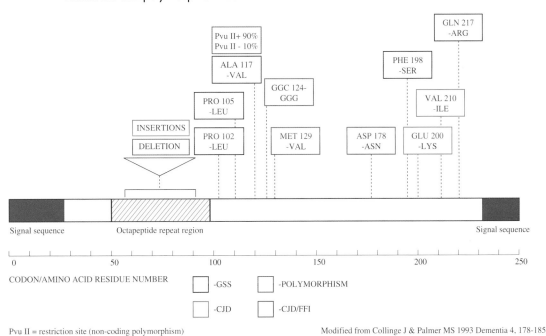

Pvu II = restriction site (non-coding polymorphism)

Modified from Collinge J & Palmer MS 1993 Dementia 4, 178-185

Note: The signal sequences are cleaved during maturation of the protein. The octa-peptide repeat region may be polymorphic as a result of a deletion (which is not associated with disease) or multiple (4-9) insertions, which are. In each case the second named amino acid (*eg* LEU 102 = Leucine codon 102) or base sequence (*eg* GGG 124) is that found in the patient with familial disease. The phenotype resulting from the mutation at codon 178 (asparagine) presents either as CJD or FFI (fatal familial insomnia) depending on the polymphorhism at codon 129 - methionine determines FFI and valine CJD. Valine 129 homozygosity also occurs in a disproportionately large number of hGH-related iatrogenic CJD patients.

infection for man and it is concluded there is no epidemiological association between the two diseases. One of the most compelling arguments to support this contention is that CJD exists in Australia and New Zealand at the same incidence as elsewhere in the world, but no scrapie (or BSE) exists in those countries because of rigidly enforced import controls. CJD is predominantly (85% of cases) a sporadic disease but about 14% of cases are familial and associated with mutations in the *PrP* gene (Figure 1.7). Less than 1% are iatrogenic (accidentally transmitted from man to man as a result of medical or surgical procedures).

Cases of iatrogenic CJD have been recorded in the USA, Great Britain (GB), France, Australia, Brazil and New Zealand as a result of the treatment of patients many years earlier with growth hormone (hGH) or gonadotrophin (hPG) derived from human pituitary glands. In the UK, treatment with hGH ceased in 1985 and safe recombinant hormones are now used. A few cases have also occurred following ocular surgery (1 case) or neurosurgery which employed biological materials from human cadavers, or following invasive neurological procedures. These are tragic and rare occurrences and controls are in place to prevent any recurrence.

In sporadic CJD, differences in the gene sequence, whilst not responsible for the disease, may modify its clinical expression (phenotype). A good example of this is the codon 129 polymorphism of the human *PrP* gene which codes either for the amino acids methionine (M) or valine (V). All three possible genotypes (MM, MV and VV) exist in the healthy, normal population without effect; in Caucasians the proportions in populations are 37%, 51% and 12% respectively. In most human patients with sporadic CJD and in patients developing CJD after iatrogenic exposure to CJD there is an excess of homozygous genotypes (MM or VV). Heterozygosity seems to confer a measure of resistance following iatrogenic exposure to CJD agent. Furthermore, in combination with other mutations in the *PrP* gene, the phenotypic expression of disease may be manifested in very different ways, depending on which of the two homozygous forms exists.

CJD, in contrast to kuru, presents as a rapidly progressive dementia terminating in death, typically in 3 - 6 months from the onset of clinical signs.

Dementia is often accompanied or followed by one or more of the following: cerebellar signs; myoclonic jerking movements; cortical blindness; akinetic mutism; pyramidal, extrapyramidal and cerebellar signs. The electroencephalogram (EEG) may be pathognomic with repetitive, triphasic complexes occurring at a frequency of 1-2/Hz. Translated into simple language this means patients show loss of memory and mental faculties which may include impairment of speech, balance and vision. Continuous jerking movements and incoordination of movement often develop, patients become entirely dependent upon nursing assistance and eventually die. Absence of a major sign complicates the clinical diagnosis. The spectrum of clinical signs is broad and overlaps that of GSS (see below) and some other dementias. Except for some iatrogenic cases incubation period is not an appropriate term to use in this disease, because the date of exposure to the infectious pathogen is not known if this indeed occurs. In iatrogenic cases it ranges from 18 months, for central exposures, up to 25 years for peripheral exposures. Apart from these cases the age of onset ranges from 50 to 75 years. Atypical forms of disease occur with significant deviations from these clinical features, *eg* durations ranging from 5 to 11 years and occurrence in patients outside the usual age range. CJD has a worldwide distribution at an annual incidence of about one case per two million. Clusters of cases occur, notably in Israel, Chile and Czechoslovakia, but these are due to familial forms of the disease.

Gerstmann-Sträussler-Scheinker syndrome (GSS) was first described in 1936 and is inherited as an autosomal dominant disease. The clinical signs overlap with those of CJD and kuru. The disease is familial, affects adults between 35 and 55 years and has a long clinical duration from 2 to 10 years. Spinocerebellar signs often precede dementia. GSS is extremely rare and affects about one patient per 10-100 million per year.

PrP gene mutations in CJD, GSS and Fatal Familial Insomnia (FFI) Recent research has established a connection between mutations in the *PrP* gene and the occurrence of familial CJD and GSS (Figure 1.7 and see para 3.2). Furthermore polymorphisms in the *PrP* gene, detected by sequencing the gene in affected patients, may also alter the clinical expression of disease, for example the age of onset and duration, not to mention particular combinations of signs, or absence of particular signs. One *PrP* gene mutation (codon 178) in combination with one or other polymorphism at codon 129, results in either CJD or fatal familial insomnia (FFI). It seems that whilst both are diseases requiring the presence of the codon 178 mutant allele, the phenotype expressed (CJD or FFI) is dependent upon the particular alleles of codon 129 expressed in the patient. The distinction between CJD/GSS variants and other dementias is blurred, but with increasing experience and knowledge of the *PrP* genotypes, in-depth analysis of the clinical signs and detailed neuropathology (including PrP distribution), it may be possible to classify these diseases with increasing confidence.

Animal TSEs

Scrapie in sheep has a worldwide distribution but is notably absent in Australia, New Zealand and some countries of South America and Europe (Table 1.1). Most breeds and both sexes are affected and the age of peak incidence is about 3½ years. The onset of disease is insidious and frequently inconspicuous, though clear enough to permit a diagnosis by the experienced observer. The fleece may be harsh to handle, exercise tolerance is reduced, the gait unsteady and water metabolism altered so that sheep drink small quantities frequently. They may also urinate abnormally, voiding small quantities of urine, and rumination may be reduced. Rubbing the poll and buttocks in response to pruritus is common, though does not occur in all cases. In Iceland for example, in the classical rida area (rida is the Icelandic name for scrapie) pruritus was hardly seen at all.

Behavioural changes are exhibited in several ways. Animals may be more nervous or aggressive and may seek separation from the rest of the flock. Hypersensitivity to sound or movement may occur and there may be muscular twitches or tremor - hence the origin of the French word for scrapie, la tremblante. Loss of wool by rubbing and nibbling are typical features coupled, in the pre-terminal phase, with loss of condition. Rubbing the back

commonly stimulates a nibble reflex.

Ataxia (incoordination), especially of the hind limbs, is a major feature and may sometimes be accompanied by a tendency to move at the trot (hence trotting disease - Traberkrankheit in German), or to hop like a rabbit. A recently described feature in Shetland sheep in Shetland, is sudden death with characteristic pathology on *post mortem* examination. It is not known if these cases exhibit clinical signs of scrapie.

The full range of clinical signs are not shown by all sheep and there may be differences, subtle or otherwise, between scrapie in different breeds and countries. There can also be a change with time; for example in Iceland, rida now frequently presents with pruritus, whereas previously it did not do so. Studies have not been done to relate the range of clinical signs with known variables, such as the strains of agent involved and the *PrP/Sip* genotype of the host (see para 3.1).

Following the advent of BSE there has been no recorded change in the age of onset, clinical signs or duration of clinical scrapie in either sheep or goats. There is some evidence of an increased incidence of scrapie in sheep, but the true incidence is unknown as there have been no valid surveys, nor is there a surveillance system to record all cases or a representative sample. The EU Directive 91/68, which made scrapie a notifiable disease throughout the Union from 1 January 1993, also does not provide a means of estimating the incidence as individual cases are not subject to laboratory confirmation once a flock has been shown to be infected.

Scrapie in goats is similar to scrapie in sheep, although goats are generally less inclined to rub against fixed objects and instead scratch vigorously with horns or hind feet.

BSE was first identified in 1986 and may have been the source of infection in all the newly recognised SEs seen in other species since then (Table 1.2). BSE seems to have originated from feed contaminated by a scrapie-like agent derived from sheep or cattle. Infectivity was present in meat and bone meal which was inadequately treated during manufacture.

Commercially induced changes in rendering of abattoir, butchers' and knackers' waste, resulting collectively from a fall in the value of tallow, a rise in the cost of energy and a need to replace old plant with safer systems not using explosive, and potentially carcinogenic, hydrocarbon solvents, was probably responsible.

BSE has been recorded in indigenous cattle only in the United Kingdom, Republic of Ireland, France, Portugal and Switzerland. It affects adult cattle of both sexes. The age of peak incidence and median incubation period is 4-5 years. Far fewer bulls than cows are affected because the number of bulls is disproportionately small due to the commercial use of artificial insemination. The signs of BSE have remained constant throughout the epidemic. Neurological signs are insidious in onset and fit into three categories:

▲ changes in sensation with hyperaesthesia (increased sensitivity) to touch or sound, excessive nose licking and teeth grinding,

▲ changes in mental status such as apprehension, frenzy and nervousness of doorways,

▲ abnormalities of posture (low head carriage, arched back, abducted, stiff, straight and straddled hind limbs) and gait (hind limb ataxia, swaying, trotting (pacing gait), hypermetria (exaggerated raising of the limbs) and falling).

There are general signs such as loss of condition and weight and in dairy cows, loss of milk yield. Unlike scrapie, pruritus is not a major feature of BSE. More recently significant deficits in rumination have been found in BSE cases. The clinical course of BSE typically lasts a few months but can extend to over a year or be as short as 2 weeks.

SE in captive wild ruminants, domestic cats and captive wild FELIDAE SE has been observed in a total of 14 exotic ruminants of six species kept in zoos or wildlife parks in England. The initial cases in four species apparently originated from the same feed source that caused disease in cattle. However, since then, some confirmed cases in greater kudu, eland and a recent initial case in the sixth species (a scimitar-horned oryx) have occurred. All the latter were born after the ruminant feed ban (which was designed to exclude infection in ruminant feed) was

introduced. However, a much wider range of captive wild ruminants and other species also consumed similar feed before the ban, but no SE has resulted. Thus different species seem to differ in their response to similar exposures.

In captive wild ruminants the clinical course is usually very short, mostly less than a week, sometimes just a few days. The shortest duration was one day (in two greater kudu) and the longest 56 days (also in a kudu). The signs are neurological, with general weight loss being prominent in eland and oryx. The neurological signs are variable but mimicked those of scrapie and BSE. They included abnormal head posture, pruritus and frequent micturition (nyala), episodic collapse (gemsbok), hypermetria, tremor, drooling and nasal discharge (eland), tremors and ataxia (oryx), lip licking, nose twitching, abnormal head carriage and tremors (greater kudu), nasal discharge and collapse (scimitar-horned oryx).

When a cat was reported in 1990 to have succumbed to feline spongiform encephalopathy (FSE), some concern was expressed by the public and some scientists. But it was already known that this species was experimentally susceptible to CJD and had been used in the USA and Czechoslovakia for investigating the human disease. To May 1994 fifty cases of FSE in domestic cats have been reported. They occurred in most parts of the British Isles except the Republic of Ireland.

One puma and four cheetahs in captivity have also succumbed though lions, tigers and other wild cats have not. Feed is the probable source of infection and in the case of the puma it was most probably uncooked central nervous tissue from cattle.

Ataxia and abnormal behaviour are consistent features in the domestic cat and altered grooming habits and hyperaesthesia occur commonly. Abnormal head posture, tremors and hyperptyalism (salivation) occur in some cases. There is difficulty in positioning for defaecation and urination, and affected animals walk with a crouching gait. Judgement of distance required for accurate jumping is impaired. Behavioural changes include unusual aggression, or timidity with hiding.

In captive wild FELIDAE ataxia is a consistent feature. A single affected puma showed a fine whole body tremor. One cheetah had central ataxia described as balancing problems and another was hyperaesthetic.

Chronic wasting disease (CWD) is a rare disease and affects only CERVIDAE (deer family) and has not been observed outside North America. Surveillance of deer in GB has shown no evidence of an unknown neurological condition, or of spongiform encephalopathy. Weight loss and emaciation are constant signs in CWD-affected deer species, their crosses, and elk. Pruritus never occurs in CWD. Other signs differ in the frequency of their occurrence. Changes in behaviour consistently occur in deer and include decreased interactions with herd mates, changes in response to attendants and periods of somnolence. Hyperexcitability and hind limb ataxia are only rarely seen in deer. In elk, behavioural signs are not consistently seen but hyperaesthesia and increased nervousness do occur. Polydypsia, with abnormal drinking behaviour and polyuria, are common in deer, much less so in elk. In some 15% of cases in deer the oesophagus is dilated, filled with water and ruminal contents which are regurgitated. This can lead to fatal aspiration pneumonia.

Transmissible mink encephalopathy (TME) is a rare disease of farmed mink. Some outbreaks have had an exceptionally high mortality. The disease has never been reported in the UK and most incidents have been in North America, though a few have been reported from some parts of northern Europe. The origin of the disease is presumed to be sheep infected with scrapie, uncooked tissues from which are fed to the mink. Experimental induction of TME by feeding scrapie-infected tissues has not been successful. However, inoculation does result in disease, but with an incubation period many months longer than in the natural incidents.

In some instances in North America, sheep material was not fed, so it has been postulated that in cattle in the United States (US) there may rarely be a sub-clinical form of transmissible spongiform encephalopathy and this may be the source. In one particular incident 'downer cows' formed a high proportion of the feed for mink, although it should be noted that such feed has been used on many mink farms without causing disease. Experimentally one isolate of TME can be

transmitted to cattle and re-isolated in mink, and BSE can be transmitted to mink by inoculation or feeding.

The clinical onset of TME is subtle and insidious. Hyperaesthesia, hyperexcitability and increased aggression are common clinical signs. Affected mink show frenzied behaviour and attack when provoked. Loud noises produce an exaggerated startle response. Mink, usually clean animals, become careless with defaecation and are reluctant to climb for their feed placed on the cage top. Ataxia develops, the head posture is low and the tail is elevated over the back like that of a squirrel. A creeping gait develops, circling and body tremors occur and blindness is common. Compulsive biting of the body leads to severe mutilation especially of the tail. Objects, or the cage, are bitten too with compulsive 'holding on' *eg* to a pencil held in a gloved hand from which the mink can be suspended. Death occurs after a few weeks of progressive deterioration but may occur in a week or less. Experimental BSE in mink results in neurological signs but they are different from those of TME.

1.25 *Summary and conclusions*

In conclusion the TSEs are fatal, neurological diseases predominantly of adults. All the TSEs show pathological accumulation of PrP. The clinical signs for each species are generally distinctive enough to arouse the suspicion of spongiform encephalopathy as a cause. However, within species there can be variation, for example kuru and iatrogenic CJD resulting from peripheral exposure present usually as cerebellar ataxias and in contrast to sporadic CJD, dementia is a late developing sign. In BSE the signs are remarkably consistent in experimental and natural disease and over the period of the epidemic. Natural scrapie has a wider variation of signs and differs in detail between sheep and goats. Host genes, particularly the *PrP* gene, probably play an important role in all the TSEs, but only in some does genetic variation occur which directly affects the development and incubation period of disease. Some of the TSEs result from natural (scrapie) or man-made exposure (BSE, TME and kuru) directly or indirectly from infected hosts (scrapie) or via feed (BSE and TME).

Some species appear to be dead-end hosts for disease (mink for TME, humans for kuru, perhaps cattle for BSE) whereas, in others, maternal and horizontal transmission account for their endemic occurrence, in the case of scrapie, over centuries. Diagnosis can be made morphologically or by detection of PrP^{Sc}. If the genomes of the agent could be found it would probably revolutionise diagnostic and control methods to the great benefit of human and animal health. Many researchers expect the genome to be nucleic acid but none has been identified and some researchers think that the infective agent contains no nucleic acid at all but is solely protein. This has led to another form of classification - the prion diseases - though many scientists have great difficulty with the concept of a replicating protein anomaly.

Reading list

AGUZZI A, BRANDNER S, SURE U, RÜEDI D AND ISENMANN S. (1994) Transgenic and knock-out mice: models of neurological disease. Brain. Path. *4*, 3-20.

AUSTIN A R AND SIMMONS M M. (1993) Reduced rumination in bovine spongiform encephalopathy and scrapie. Vet. Rec. *132*, 324-5.

BAKER H AND RIDLEY R M. (1991) Human spongiform encephalopathy. Chemistry and Industry. 4 March 1991, 163-168. (A concise account for the layman).

BENNETT A D, BIRKETT C R AND BOSTOCK C J. (1992) Molecular biology of scrapie-like agents. Rev. sci. tech. Off. int. Epiz. *11*, 569-603.

BOVINE SPONGIFORM ENCEPHALOPATHY. RECENT RESEARCH AND CONTROL OF THE DISEASE. (1994) Editors R Bradley and R D Politiek. Livestock Production Science Special Issue. *38*, pp 59.

BROWN P. (1994) Infectious cerebral amyloidoses: Creutzfeldt-Jakob disease and Gerstmann-Sträussler-Scheinker syndrome. Neurol. Dis. Ther. *22*, 353-375.

BROWN P, CATHALA F, RAUBERTAS R F, GAJDUSEK D C AND CASTAIGNE P. (1987) The epidemiology of Creutzfeldt-Jakob disease: Conclusion of a 15 year investigation in France and review of the world literature. Neurology *37*, 895-904.

BRUCE M E. (1993) Scrapie strain variation and mutation. Br. Med. Bull. *49*, 822-838.

BÜELER H, AGUZZI A, SAILER A, GREINER R-A, AUTENRIED P, AGUET M AND WEISSMANN C. (1993) Mice devoid of PrP are resistant to scrapie. Cell *73*, 1339-1347.

CAMERON E R, HARVEY M J A AND ONIONS D E. (1994) Transgenic science. Br. vet. J. *150*, 9-24.

CAUGHEY B AND RAYMOND G J. (1993) Sulfated polyanion inhibition of scrapie-associated PrP accumulation in cultured cells. J. Virol. *67*, 643-650.

CHESEBRO B AND CAUGHEY B. (1993) Scrapie agent replication without the prion protein? Curr. Biol. *3*, 696-698.

CLARK A M AND MOAR J A E. (1992) Scrapie: A clinical assessment. Vet. Rec. *130*, 377-378.

COLLINGE J AND PALMER M S. (1993) Prion diseases in humans and their relevance to other neurodegenerative diseases. Dementia *4*, 178-185.

DARNELL J, LODISH H AND BALTIMORE D. (1990) Molecular Cell Biology, 2nd ed. Chapter 2, Molecules and cells, pp 14-54. Scientific American Books, Freeman, New York.

GOLDFARB L G, BROWN P AND GAJDUSEK D C. (1992) The molecular genetics of human transmissible spongiform encephalopathy. In: Prion Diseases of Humans and Animals. Editors S B Prusiner, J Collinge, J Powell and B Anderton. Ellis Horwood, Chichester, pp 139-153.

HUNTER N AND HOPE J. (1991) The genetics of scrapie susceptibility in sheep (and its implications for BSE). In: Breeding for Disease Resistance in Farm Animals. Editors J B Owen and R F E Axford. Chapter 19. CAB International, Wallingford, pp 329-344.

KIMBERLIN R H. (1990) Unconventional "slow" viruses. In: Topley and Wilson's Principles of Bacteriology, Virology and Immunity. 8th Edition. Editors L H Collier and M C Timbury. Edward Arnold, London, *4*, 671-693.

KIMBERLIN R H. (1992) Bovine spongiform encephalopathy. Rev. sci. tech. Off. int. Epiz. *11,* 347-390.

KIRKWOOD J K AND CUNNINGHAM A A. (1994) Spongiform encephalopathy in captive wild animals in Britain: epidemiological observations. Vet. Rec. Submitted.

KRETZSCHMAR H A. (1993) Human prion diseases (spongiform encephalopathies). Arch. Virol. (Suppl) *7,* 261-293.

ÖZEL M AND DIRINGER H. (1994) Small virus-like structure in fractions from scrapie hamster brain. Lancet *343,* 894-895.

PALMER M S AND COLLINGE J. (1993) Mutations and polymorphisms in the prion protein gene. Human Mutation *2,* 168-173.

PAN K -M, BALDWIN M, NGUYEN J, GASSET M, SERBAN A, GROTH D, MEHLHORN I, HUANG Z, FLETTERICK R J, COHEN F E AND PRUSINER S B. (1993) Conversion of α-helices into β-sheets features in the formation of the scrapie prion proteins. Proc. Natl. Acad. Sci. USA *90,* 10962-10966.

PARRY H B. (1983) Scrapie disease in sheep. Historical, clinical, epidemiological, pathological and practical aspects of the natural disease. Editor D R Oppenheimer. Academic Press, London, pp 192.

PRION DISEASES OF HUMANS AND ANIMALS. (1992) Editors S B Prusiner, J Collinge, J Powell, B Anderton. Ellis Horwood, Chichester, pp 583.

PRUSINER S B. (1993) Genetic and infectious prion diseases. Arch. Neurol. *50,* 1129-1153.

SAFAR J, ROLLER P P, GAJDUSEK D C AND GIBBS Jr C J. (1993) Conformational transitions, dissociation and unfolding of scrapie amyloid (prion) protein. J. Biol. Chem. *268,* 20276-20284.

SAILER A, BÜELER H, FRASER M, AGUZZI A AND WEISSMANN C. (1994) No propagation of prions in mice devoid of PrP. Cell *77,* 967-968.

SIGURDSSON B. (1954) Rida, a chronic encephalitis of sheep. With general remarks on infections which develop slowly and some of their special characteristics. Br. Vet. J. *110,* 341-355.

STAHL N, BALDWIN M A, HECKER R, PAN K M, BURLINGAME A L AND PRUSINER S B. (1992) Glycosylinositol phospholipid anchors of the scrapie and cellular prion proteins contain sialic acid. Biochem. *31,* 5043-5053.

TARABOULOS A, JENDROSKA K, SERBAN D, YANG S L, DeARMOND S J AND PRUSINER S B. (1992) Regional mapping of prion proteins in brain. Proc. Natl. Acad. Sci. USA *89,* 7620-7624.

TRANSMISSIBLE SPONGIFORM ENCEPHALOPATHIES OF ANIMALS. (1992) Editors R Bradley and D Matthews. OIE Scientific and Technical Review *11,* pp 634.

TRANSMISSIBLE SPONGIFORM ENCEPHALOPATHIES. SCRAPIE, BSE AND RELATED DISORDERS. (1991) Editor B W Chesebro. Current Topics in Microbiology and Immunology. Springer-Verlag, Berlin, pp 288.

TYRRELL D A J. (1992) An overview of bovine spongiform encephalopathy (BSE) in Britain. Dev. Biol. Standard *76,*275-284.

WELLS, G A H, SCOTT A C, JOHNSON C T, GUNNING R F, HANCOCK R D, JEFFREY M, DAWSON M AND BRADLEY R. (1987) A novel progressive spongiform encephalopathy in cattle. Vet. Rec. *121,* 419-420.

WESTAWAY D, DeARMOND S J, CAYETANO-CANLAS J, GROTH D, FOSTER D, YANG S L, TORCHIA M, CARLSON G A AND PRUSINER S B. (1994) Degeneration of skeletal muscle peripheral nerves, and the central nervous system in transgenic mice overexpressing wild-type prion proteins. Cell *76,* 117-129.

WILESMITH J W, HOINVILLE L J, RYAN J B M AND SAYERS A R. (1992) Bovine spongiform encephalopathy: aspects of the clinical picture and analyses of possible changes 1986-1990. Vet. Rec. *130,* 197-201.

WYATT J M, PEARSON G P AND GRUFFYDD-JONES T J. (1993) Feline spongiform encephalopathy. Feline Practice *21,* 7-11.

XI Y G, INGROSSO L, LADOGANA A, MASULLO C AND POCCHIARI M. (1992) Amphotericin B treatment dissociates *in vivo* replication of the scrapie agent from PrP accumulation. Nature *356,* 598-601.

31

Epidemiology

2.1 *Scrapie history and epidemiology*

Scrapie is the oldest known transmissible spongiform encephalopathy and is the archetype for all members of this group of diseases. The earliest reports go back to the early part of the eighteenth century. The disease is known by a number of other names (goggles, rubbers, shakers, scratchie, cuddie trot) in Great Britain, la tremblante in France, Traberkrankheit in Germany, rida in Iceland and súrlókór (brushing disease) in Hungary.

In the period 1700-1880 scrapie was a well recognised disease in western Europe as far east as the Danube valley (1820-1880) and as far south as Spain (1750-1880). Severe epidemics were encountered in England and Wales (1750-1820) and Germany (1780-1820). Except in Scotland the disease declined to insignificant levels in the period 1880-1910 after which it has increased in Great Britain and France (since 1980) and has appeared in several other countries (*eg* Italy, Spain, Switzerland, The Netherlands), some (*eg* Iceland, Cyprus, Germany and Norway) by importation. Outside Europe the disease occurs in North America, southern Africa, India, Japan; has been eradicated from Australia and New Zealand (by compulsory slaughter (with compensation) of imported sheep and flockmates shortly after release from quarantine) and does not appear to exist in Denmark, Argentina or Uruguay and probably many other countries.

The incidence of scrapie in affected countries is rarely published officially even where it is compulsorily notifiable. The Office International des Epizooties (OIE) receives annual reports from their Member countries on whether or not the disease occurs. Awareness is extremely high in the big sheep rearing countries like Argentina, Australia and New Zealand where occurrence would have serious consequences for trade in sheep and sheep products. In other countries the disease may be concealed since, if a diagnosis is made, a flock may be blighted (*ie* the sale value of breeding stock may be reduced). However, the disease probably occurs at a moderate incidence in Great Britain and at a lower incidence in Northern Ireland, the Republic of Ireland and perhaps in most other countries in Europe and North America where its presence has been reported.

The first microscopic lesions to be described in natural scrapie were vacuoles in the perikaryon of ventral horn cells of the spinal cord in the late nineteenth century. Nowadays clinical diagnosis is usually confirmed by microscopic examination of the brain. In earlier times scrapie was suspected to be a hereditary disease because of its familial pattern of occurrence, but numerous other causes were considered, including sarcocystis infection.

Cuillé and Chelle, working in Toulouse in France, were the first to successfully transmit scrapie to sheep by intra-ocular inoculation of CNS material from clinically affected sheep. The incubation period was 14-22 months. Later, in 1942, Chelle first reported natural scrapie in the goat and Wood and Done did likewise for captive moufflon (wild mountain sheep) in 1992. In the period 1946-1950 Gordon, Greig and Wilson demonstrated the resistance of scrapie agent to formalin and to boiling, and showed that it would pass filters of 410nm, thus indicating the small size of the agent responsible. Wilson and his co-workers also transmitted the disease in series from sheep to sheep for nine passages, and thus showed that the agent could replicate itself. In 1959 Stamp and colleagues transmitted scrapie from sheep to sheep using brain, spleen, lymph node and cerebrospinal fluid.

In 1961 Chandler first transmitted scrapie to mice, thus providing researchers with a relatively inexpensive experimental model but only for some purposes. Golden hamsters were developed later as a model for molecular studies on the agents. Dickinson showed that scrapie was transmitted from ewe to lamb. He also developed genetically different inbred lines of mice which he subsequently used with Bruce and Fraser to demonstrate agent strain variation, agent mutation and how the agent strain interacts with the host genotype. This interaction determines the incubation period and lesion profile in the brain.

Dickinson with Outram also proposed the virino hypothesis of agent structure. Kimberlin and Walker established the concept of clinical target areas in scrapie infection. These are areas of the brain in which infection must replicate for clinical disease to develop. They also extended considerably the knowledge of scrapie agent strains and the factors controlling the species barrier.

The commonly accepted view is that scrapie is an infectious and contagious disease and import controls for live sheep are based on this idea. A notable exception to this view was held by H B Parry who, as a result of many years of research, was convinced that the disease was hereditary, being caused by an autosomal recessive gene, and that contagion was not the usual means of spread. We now know that there is a gene *(Sip)* which controls the incubation period length and under some conditions, the presence of an allele of this gene can determine whether disease occurs during the life of a sheep. This gene and its relation to the prion protein *(PrP)* gene are discussed elsewhere in this report. Scrapie is experimentally transmissible to other species. It has not been shown to occur in genetically predisposed sheep without exposure to the infection. The agent is extraordinarily resistant to inactivation by physical and chemical treatments which are effective for inactivating conventional viruses.

Pattison, with his co-workers, demonstrated that goats were universally susceptible to experimental scrapie and showed that placenta from Swaledale ewes with scrapie was infective for both sheep and goats even by feeding, thus establishing a possible source and route of infection to explain why scrapie was an endemic disease.

Hadlow recognised the pathological resemblance of scrapie to kuru and suggested to Gadjusek that transmission studies using primates should be attempted to establish whether or not kuru could be transmitted. This was subsequently achieved by Gibbs, Gajdusek and colleagues and was reported in 1968. Later they succeeded in transmitting CJD too. Hadlow conducted a comprehensive set of studies on the pathogenesis of natural scrapie in Suffolk sheep. His results were used to plan measures to protect animals and humans from exposure to BSE agents before the results of tests of the infectivity of bovine tissues were available. Meanwhile Dickinson, Kimberlin and colleagues had established the essential features of the dynamics and control of agent replication in different tissues which determined the pathogenesis of experimental scrapie in mice. Following inoculation there was a 'zero phase' during which infection was undetectable. Multiplication of the agent was detected first in the lymphoreticular system. Development of disease depended on later invasion of the thoracic spinal cord (probably via the splanchnic nerve), and spread of agent to many parts of the CNS, particularly the brain. The *Sinc* gene seemed to control neuroinvasion and the rate of spread, multiplication and progression of the agent in the CNS.

In summary it is generally accepted that scrapie is transmitted in family lines in flocks by some form of maternal transmission, possibly to the pre-implantation embryo and later via placental infection. This same source is presumed to account for at least some horizontal (lateral) transmission to flockmates, either directly (by consumption) or indirectly from a contaminated environment. Horizontal transmission to other ewe lines is one reason why scrapie is an endemic disease and why it is so difficult to eradicate. Following infection there is a zero phase lasting until sheep are at least 8 months old. Infection is undetectable by bioassay in mice in any tissue during this period. Subsequently replication occurs in lymphoreticular tissues and the CNS is invaded, typically around 2 years of age. This is followed by further replication, and lesions and clinical signs develop typically at 3½ years.

The epidemiology of natural scrapie has a much longer history than that of BSE, and has been more difficult to investigate. The major milestones have been given above. Study of experimental scrapie in sheep, goats, mice and hamsters has enormously advanced our understanding of the agent, the pathogenesis and the control of disease occurrence, but a better epidemiological understanding of natural scrapie is needed so that improved control measures can be developed and their effects monitored.

2.2 *Bovine spongiform encephalopathy*

By contrast with scrapie this disease has only been recognised since the mid 1980s, and the story of how the first cases occurred in 1985 and 1986 throughout the UK has been described in detail. The first cases were recognised to be a spongiform encephalopathy resembling scrapie. A systematic epidemiological study was set, up based on diagnosis by clinical examination and confirmation by neuropathological examination of the brain stem. The results were collated and analysed at the Central Veterinary Laboratory (CVL), Weybridge. It was established that the disease was not associated with a range of possible risk factors. Factors eliminated included the importation of animals or animal products, vaccines, pharmaceutical products, agricultural chemicals or direct contact with sheep. The only common factors in herds with confirmed BSE cases were the use of proprietary feeds or protein supplements containing ruminant-derived protein, usually in the form of meat and bone meal. This was produced in part by rendering waste tissues, including CNS, from sheep and cattle. These tissues were derived largely from abattoirs and butchers.

Meat and bone meal supplements were fed mostly to dairy calves and so had a particular impact on dairy herds and much less effect on beef suckler herds. The cumulative dairy herd and suckler herd incidences to August 1994 are 51.9% and 13.7%

respectively. The modal incubation period cannot be precisely determined because the time of exposure is not accurately known. However, because most exposures were in calves it is likely to approximate to the modal age of onset. This is 4 - 5 years (range 20 months to 18 years). Adult exposures are presumed to be responsible for disease in at least some of the older animals. The incubation period distribution has been estimated with apparently sufficient accuracy to provide estimates of the future numbers of cases for budgetary purposes. At present the risk of exposure appears to have been greatest for calves. This is consistent with the past inclusion rates of meat and bone meal in calf and adult rations. Cohort analyses, which represent part of the continuous epidemiological monitoring of the epidemic, will provide a more complete understanding of the contribution from exposure in adulthood.

The outbreak probably began because scrapie agent in the brains and offals of infected (but not necessarily clinically affected) sheep was not so well inactivated in the early 1980s as it had been earlier. This was because the processing (rendering) of offal into meat and bone meal (MBM) was modified then for commercial reasons, so that hydrocarbon solvents were much less used and the additional steam treatment used to remove solvents for re-use was also omitted. It is suggested that the increasing amount of infectious bovine CNS tissues entering the rendering system from about 1984 resulted in a further increase in BSE incidence in the summer of 1989, since there would no longer have been a species barrier to infection of cattle via feed contaminated with bovine tissue (Figure 2.1).

Epidemiological, pathological, transmission, statistical population genetic studies and molecular genetic studies of the *PrP* gene in cattle have shown that host genetic variation in the *PrP* or other bovine genes is not a major factor in the occurrence of BSE. Therefore it is postulated that in the UK the sporadic incidence of BSE is due to a random low dose exposure, possibly due to the relatively low concentration of 'packets' of infection sufficient to cause disease in many feed batches. As the epidemic progressed and recycling of infected cattle offals became dominant it seems that the number of 'packets' increased, with little increase in agent concentration per 'packet' thus increasing the likelihood of a herd owner purchasing an infected batch. Such a scenario would suggest that the rising incidence of BSE would be accounted for by new infections in previously uninfected herds rather than an increase in cases in herds already affected. This fits the epidemiological findings of a low and relatively constant within-herd incidence of around 3%, the risk of herd infection being greater with increasing herd size and 70% of affected herds having three cases of BSE or less since 1988. These data also support the view of a common source epidemic of a non-contagious agent, rather than a propagating epidemic of a contagious agent.

There have been no changes in either the clinical presentation or the neuropathology of BSE over the course of the epidemic. This is consistent with the hypothesis that a single agent strain is involved in all incidents. This is also borne out by agent strain typing studies. A limited number of BSE isolates are being strain-typed by their lesion profile and incubation period length in genetically different inbred mouse lines. The results confirm those of

field epidemiology and show that BSE from successive years since late 1987 is due to the same strain and is indistinguishable from the isolates obtained from the other species recently affected with SE. BSE has been confirmed in virtually all breeds of cattle in GB. Within dairy breeds the number of confirmed cases is directly proportional to the number of animals in each breed in the country. Thus Holstein Friesians, being the predominant dairy breed in the UK, are the most frequently affected.

Control

Control measures are necessary for public health and animal health reasons, the former because the BSE agent may be a human pathogen and the latter because the disease causes economic loss to the industry as a result of loss of public confidence, reduced international trade and illness and death of affected animals. Because of self-inflicted injury especially as a result of falling this disease also creates animal welfare problems. Since the epidemic was identified measures have been taken

Figure 2.1 Epidemic curve. Confirmed cases of BSE plotted by month and year of clinical onset

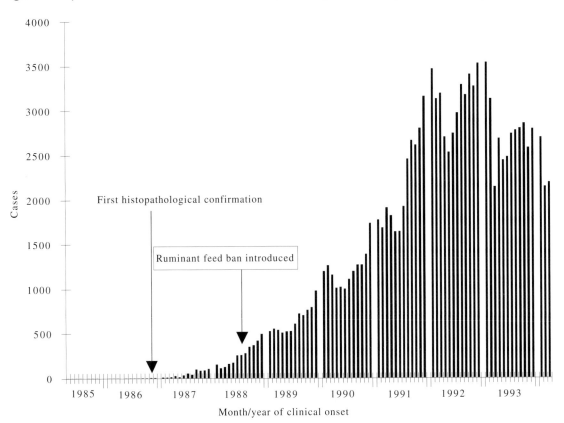

Cases recorded prior to the first histopathological confirmation were identifed by retrospective examination of clinical histories. Data valid to end of March 1994. Produced 13 September 1994.

to control it in Great Britain. In Northern Ireland similar measures were introduced a few weeks or months later. In GB, since 21 June 1988 BSE has been compulsorily notifiable. In GB, since 8 August 1988 suspected animals, believed by MAFF veterinary officers to have BSE, are compulsorily slaughtered and the carcases of all such cases are completely destroyed, virtually all of them by incineration since 1991. As an extra precautionary measure and on the advice of the Southwood Working Party, milk from suspect animals is prohibited from sale or use to feed man or animals except, for welfare reasons, the dam's own calf. It seemed logical to recommend this since complete destruction of the whole carcase of suspect cases had been recommended earlier. The feeding of cattle with ruminant-derived protein (other than milk protein) was banned from 18 July 1988 in GB and from January 1989 in Northern Ireland. The number of confirmed cases of BSE almost doubled (200%) from 1988 to 1989 but thereafter the rate of rise from year to year progressively diminished to 150% of the 1991 figure in 1992 and fell to 92% of the 1992 figure in 1993 (Figure 2.2).

To avoid exposure of other species to BSE agent, specified bovine offals (SBO) (*ie* brain, spinal cord, tonsil, thymus, spleen and intestine (from

duodenum to rectum) from cattle over 6 months of age* slaughtered in Great Britain) are not permitted to be fed to man (since 13 November 1989 in England and Wales and from January 1990 in Scotland and Northern Ireland). Since 25 September 1990 the SBO or protein derived from them may not be fed to any animal or bird in the UK. These tissues were identified as being those most likely to harbour the BSE agent during the incubation period by analogy with the data from bioassay of tissues from goats and Suffolk sheep naturally infected with scrapie. They are removed from carcases, dyed and stored separately from other offals in dedicated marked containers. They are either incinerated or rendered, and if rendered the protein products are safely disposed of by incineration or licensed burial. No protein product from these offals is permitted to enter any food or feed chain.

---

* Following the experimental challenge of cattle with brain from confirmed cases of BSE, infectivity (but not disease) was found in the distal ileum (small intestine closest to the large intestine) in calves 10 months of age, 6 months after dosing. Consequently Ministers decided, for reasons of extreme prudence, to extend the SBO ban for intestine and thymus only, to calves of any age, killed for human consumption.

Figure 2.2 Number of suspected cases of BSE in successive calving seasons

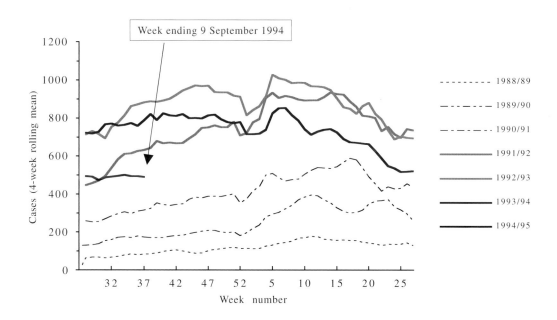

The rolling mean is the mean of suspects reported in Great Britain over a 4 - week period. Weekly fluctuations are therefore eliminated, thus facilitating comparison of one year with another.

Because of the long incubation period of experimental BSE in mice, the SBO ban had to be introduced before the results of research on the properties of the BSE agent and its tissue distribution could be completed. The ban was devised on the basis of research done many years earlier on the pathogenesis of experimental scrapie in mice and natural scrapie in sheep and goats. The expectation was that the infectivity of tissues from cows with BSE would be no greater. However it was realised that the assumptions made on the basis of natural scrapie needed to be checked, because the tissue distribution of BSE infectivity might have differed from that of scrapie. It was also important to recognise that studies could initially only be done with tissues from clinically affected animals, not from those incubating the disease. This was because in BSE there appeared to be no maternal transmission, the within-herd incidence was usually very low and there was no way of identifying infected animals during the incubation period. Thus to determine the infectivity of tissues during the incubation period, cattle would have to be experimentally infected orally with infective brain in sufficient dose to cause disease. Account would also have to be taken of variation in the *PrP* genotype of the experimental animals in case this

caused variation in the incubation period of disease. These factors delayed the initiation of the appropriate 'pathogenesis' study in cattle. The results of research on the infectivity of tissues from terminal cases of BSE are emerging (see para 5.12) and the cattle pathogenesis study is well underway.

Maternal transmission

A number of approaches have been and are being made to detect maternal transmission at the earliest opportunity, should it have occurred. One approach has been to compare the observed incidence in the offspring of cases with that expected from the food - borne source. The expected incidence has been estimated using four methods. The first two methods are based on a probability model. The first uses a 'whole herd' approach in which the population of animals is considered as 'one herd'. The second uses an individual herd approach whereby the animals are considered as being aggregated into individual herds. The third method calculates the expected number of cases from the number of offspring recorded on the main BSE epidemiological database. The fourth method calculates the expected number of cases from the number of offspring of cases which can be expected

Table 2.1 Change in age specific incidences of confirmed cases of BSE in home-bred herds from 1989-1994

Age of onset of BSE cases (years)	% Incidence of BSE in home-bred herds					
	1989	1990	1991	1992	1993	1994*
2 - 3	0.07	0.07	**0.02**	**0.02**	**0.01**	**0.00**
3 - 4	0.79	1.31	1.87	**0.65**	**0.44**	**0.04**
4 - 5	3.40	3.93	5.75	6.71	**3.31**	**1.59**
5 - 6	3.51	3.47	3.91	6.53	8.16	**3.27**
6 - 7	1.57	2.00	1.98	2.78	5.04	4.75
7 - 8	0.43	0.70	0.90	1.03	1.66	1.72

* Data as at 1 July 1994

The ruminant protein feed ban was introduced 18 July 1988

Numbers indicate the frequency of cases in well documented herds *eg* in 1990 there were 2 cases per hundred in 6-7- year-old animals. From 1991 the frequency has been declining year by year in successive older age classes as indicated by the bold underlined figures. The cause of the decline was the prevention of new infections via feed by introduction of the ruminant feed ban in July 1988.

Data courtesy of Mr J W Wilesmith.

to have survived to adulthood. This prediction has been compared with the number of actual cases in offspring of cases. In no year has there been any excess of observed cases over those predicted, thus showing that if maternal transmission does occur, it is occurring at a very low and currently undetectable frequency. Furthermore, even if maternal transmission occurred at an incidence of 100%, it still could not sustain the epidemic because, on average, affected cattle could not produce as many offspring as there are existing cases.

Laboratory studies using mice have shown that placenta from clinically affected cattle contains no detectable infectivity (see para 5.12). As suggested by the Southwood Working Party, a large experiment to look for maternal transmission was also set up (see para 5.16). In this study 29 cases of BSE have occurred till September 1994, but because some affected calves were born before the feed ban was implemented, and all within 6 months of it, all of the cases could be a result of feed exposure. The study cannot be interpreted until the last cattle are killed in November 1996 and the data analysed. At that time it may indicate whether or not maternal transmission can occur and if it does, the frequency. However, at present it is not possible to determine that maternal transmission has

occurred, but nor can it be ruled out. However, at the worst there has not been a high incidence of maternal transmission of disease. These findings imply that, as with mink and TME, cattle may be a 'dead end' host for BSE with no natural routes of transmission of infection.

Effects of the ruminant protein ban of 18 July 1988

The epidemic curve (Figure 2.1) which plots the number of confirmed cases of BSE by the date of onset of clinical signs is the definitive method for describing the epidemic and showing any change in incidence. However, it is necessarily a retrospective representation of the epidemic (about 6 months in arrears) because of the length of the clinical period of disease and the time taken for confirmation of disease to be made and plotted on the curve. To overcome this difficulty other methods of demonstrating changes in incidence have been used. For example, an early indication that the ruminant feed ban was beginning to have an effect was seen as a reduction in the incidence of confirmed BSE in the 2- year - old age class, towards the end of 1991. This reduction was sustained and with each successive year the next oldest age class also showed a reduction in incidence (Table 2.1).

Figure 2.3 Comparison of the report rate of suspect BSE cases over 4 - week periods with that of 12 months earlier

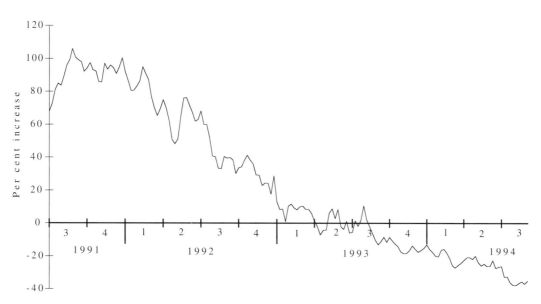

The 0 % line represents the report rate 12 months earlier. Each calendar year is divided into four quarters as indicated.

Further confidence that the feed ban has been effective is shown by the reduction in the rate of increase of reported, suspected BSE cases from the autumn of 1992. Now (9 September 1994) the number of suspect BSE cases placed under restriction is 37% below that at the same time in 1993 (Figures 2.2 and 2.3). Another way of illustrating the effectiveness of the feed ban is to compare the actual and predicted numbers of cases of BSE that would have occurred without a feed ban. The predicted data are developed from the computer simulation model, and show that there were at least 20,000 fewer cases of BSE than would have occurred in 1992 without the ban and over 30,000 fewer in 1993.

The explanation for the delayed response to the control measures is that many animals had been infected before the feed ban was introduced in July 1988 and were only revealed as clinical cases with the lapse of time because of the long incubation period of the disease. As in scrapie, there is no way of detecting, eliminating or treating infected, clinically healthy animals, so this aspect of the epidemic could not be curtailed. Continued recording of cases and analysis of the results is enabling us to refine our estimates of the incubation period. This was originally calculated to be from 2 years to at least 8 years with a log normal distribution, and is now calculated to have a median incubation time of 5 years with most cases occurring in animals between 4 and 6 years of age and does not seem to have changed significantly.

BSE in animals born after July 1988

There was surprise in some quarters that despite the imposition of the animal health controls in 1988 (ruminant feed ban) and 1990 (SBO ban for feeding to other species) 12,807 cases of BSE have been confirmed (to mid September 1994) in animals born after the 1988 ban, and this has given rise to comment. This was because it was expected that the ban could be implemented immediately, but this view did not take account of human nature and the practical difficulties involved. As nothing was done to eliminate the large amount of feed already in the distribution 'pipeline', the benefits of the ban were not instantaneous and complete. More detailed analyses have now been made which show that the

Figure 2.4 The distribution of cases of BSE (confirmed by 1st July 1994) by the month of birth

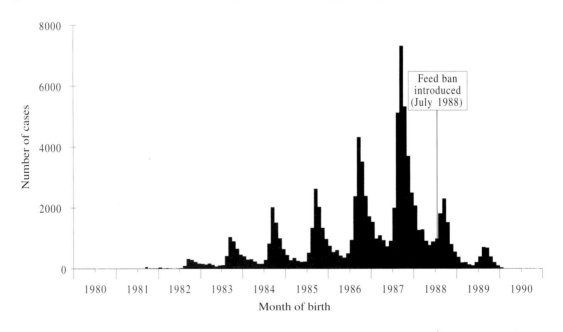

This shows the decline in the incidence from the date of implementation of the ruminant feed ban. However all the figures are interim and in particular there will be more cases in cattle born in 1989 and 1990.

Data courtesy of Dr L Hoinville.

number of confirmed cases in animals born after the ban (BAB) is much lower than expected if the epidemic had continued its previous pattern (Figure 2.4).

The majority of the BAB animals were born in the calving season following the introduction of the ban *ie* in 1988/89 (Figure 2.4). The number of cases in animals born after the ban could still rise significantly due to the high infectivity in feed manufactured up to July 1988 but consumed by cattle thereafter. Cases have also been analysed

using the results of local enquiries as to whether or not the animal might have been given contaminated feed and also whether the dam had developed BSE. The results show once again a much greater association with feed history than with the possible maternal or horizontal transmission of the disease. This all supports the deduction that this is a food-borne epidemic. However, to determine more precisely the origin of infection (feed, maternal or horizontal transmission) in the BAB animals, a case control study of animals born after October 1988 on

Figure 2.5 Variation in the species barrier with different strains of cloned scrapie agent

Incubation periods of three cloned strains of scrapie agent passaged from hamsters to mice

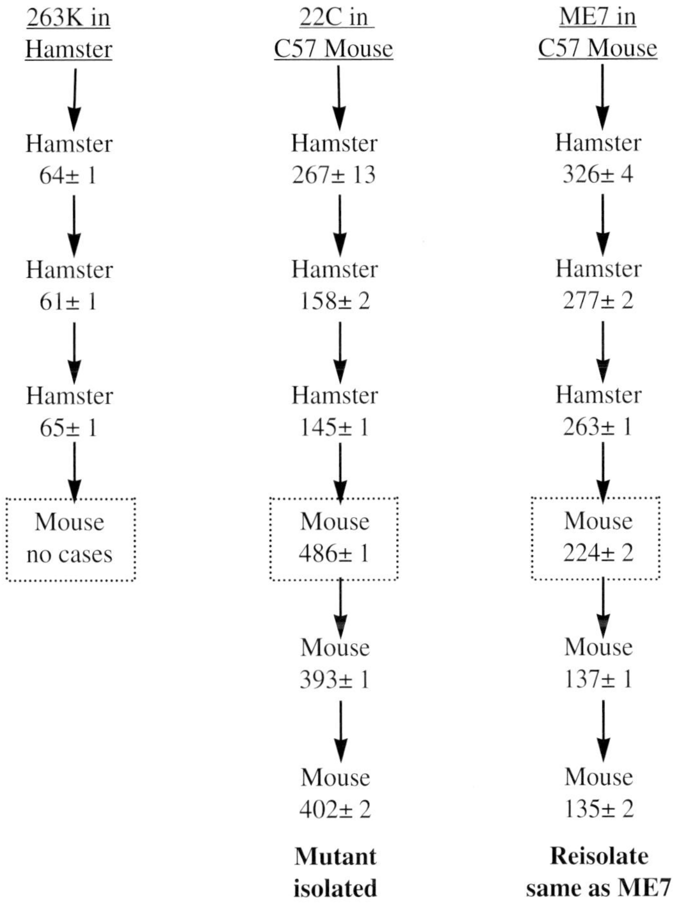

263K in Hamster	22C in C57 Mouse	ME7 in C57 Mouse
↓	↓	↓
Hamster 64± 1	Hamster 267± 13	Hamster 326± 4
↓	↓	↓
Hamster 61± 1	Hamster 158± 2	Hamster 277± 2
↓	↓	↓
Hamster 65± 1	Hamster 145± 1	Hamster 263± 1
↓	↓	↓
Mouse no cases	Mouse 486± 1	Mouse 224± 2
	↓	↓
	Mouse 393± 1	Mouse 137± 1
	↓	↓
	Mouse 402± 2	Mouse 135± 2
	Mutant isolated	**Reisolate same as ME7**

Dotted boxes signify the change of host from hamsters to mice

Homogenates of brain were passed intracerebrally in series and mean incubation periods in days ± SEM recorded.
In the 22C passage line, the strain reisolated in C57 (*Sinc* s[7]) mice was a mutant with quite different incubation period and neuropathological properties from those of 22C. In the ME7 passage line, the strain reisolated in C57 (*Sinc* s[7]) mice was identical to ME7. The 263K strain of agent did not produce clinical disease in (*Sinc* s[7]) CW mice after observation periods of up to 730 days.

Adapted from: Kimberlin RH. (1993) Bovine spongiform encephalopathy: an appraisal of the current epidemic in the United Kingdom. Intervirology *35*, 208-218.

300 farms in which home-bred animals have had BSE is in progress. This is an epidemiological study of the incidence of BSE in relation to risk factors in cattle that develop BSE and those on the same farm that do not.

Changes in the epidemic

In the early days the future size and course of the epidemic was calculated from a simple simulation model assuming no change in exposure of the cattle population with time (*ie* assuming cattle were only being exposed to sheep scrapie with no cattle-to-cattle recycling of feed-borne infection). The results were quoted in the Report of the Working Party on Spongiform Encephalopathies (Southwood Report). There has been a good deal of comment on the fact that the epidemic turned out to be much larger than predicted. However, the report pointed out that the extent of recycling, if it occurred, could not be predicted and that future estimates based on the early stages of the epidemic were bound to be unreliable if the basic epidemiological features changed, as they did. The current simulation models have the advantage of using accumulated data from the epidemic and therefore incorporate the increasing risk of infection from the recycling of infected cattle tissues. They have proved to be of practical use in predicting the resources needed to manage the epidemic. These models will be of continued value as the epidemic declines. The annual incidences of confirmed cases of BSE by year are as follows:

1988	2,184
1989	7,137
1990	14,181
1991	25,032
1992	36,677
1993	34,368
1994 (to 9 September)	14,260

It is important to realise that the epidemiological characteristics that have been established are only valid for the majority of the epidemic and for the present situation. Laboratory studies show that essentially a single strain of SE agent has caused the major part of this epidemic, which is distinct from any strain of scrapie previously known. This postulated cattle-adapted scrapie agent, derived initially from the reservoir of scrapie infection in sheep, may have been a mutant strain that arose in cattle and was preferentially selected as a result of recycling of infection between cattle via feed; this has been shown to occur with laboratory strains of rodent scrapie when transmitted parenterally to another species (Figure 2.5).

An alternative explanation is that a reservoir of BSE infection existed, and was maintained, in the British cattle population causing no more than rare cases of clinical disease (say 1 case in 10^5 adults pa). Such an infection would have been widely dispersed, naturally spread between cattle (*ie* not via feed) to maintain the endemic infection, and weakly neuroinvasive or of low neuropathogenicity to account for the low incidence of clinical disease. In this scenario, the epidemic of clinical BSE, which commenced in 1985/86, resulted from the selection by cattle of a more neuroinvasive and/or more neuropathogenic strain of agent once changes in the rendering procedures initiated a feed-borne recycling of infection in 1981/82. Thus the virulent strain of BSE agent that caused the epidemic disease would be different from its avirulent counterpart and from scrapie strains. Furthermore, the former would still be present and be maintained in the cattle population by non-feed routes of transmission if that was how it was naturally transmitted. Also, the pre-1981 prevalence of the avirulent infection could have increased because of recycling via feed.

Thus, irrespective of the origin of the epidemic, whether from sheep scrapie or pre-existing BSE infection, the development of the epidemic would have depended upon cattle-to-cattle transmission (recycling of infection) via feed. The combined effect of selection of a pathogenic strain of BSE and recycling seems the most likely explanation for the increase in incidence of BSE from July 1989 (Figure 2.1). If the occurrence of BSE had been dependent on repeated new infections of cattle from sheep-derived meat and bone meal only, the epidemic would almost certainly have been relatively insignificant. The importance of the concept that an avirulent form of BSE agent (but with the potential to evolve a virulent agent) was the original source, is that such an infection may exist in cattle elsewhere than in the UK, with the potential to cause disease if the appropriate triggering conditions were satisfied. Furthermore as the epidemic continues, if a new mutant were to emerge with a survival advantage - perhaps capable of transmitting from cow to calf - then there would be strong selection pressures for it to increase in the population, and the characteristics of the epidemic could change. So far there is no evidence for this hypothesis. However, even though such a hypothetical mutant would not be recognised until several years after its generation it could not be transmitted by feed (because of the bans in place), and maternal transmission alone is unlikely to establish the necessary net infection rate to sustain its existence (see para 2.2, sub-para maternal

transmission). Nevertheless, it is important to continue to analyse the epidemic to ensure that, as it levels off and declines, the earlier observations still apply.

BSE in other countries

Once the epidemic had been recognised and described in the UK it was obvious that BSE might occur in any country in which there was a potential link between cattle and feeds containing rendered cattle, sheep or goat tissues (*ie* ruminant derived protein) contaminated with either scrapie or BSE agents. Whether it occurred would depend on a number of factors.

Table 2.2 Number of confirmed and officially reported cases of BSE by country and year of report (to date)

Country	Year	Number	To
Great Britain[o]	1986	134,202	2 Sep 1994
Guernsey[o]	1987	496	23 Aug 1994
Northern Ireland[o]	1988	1,379	19 Aug 1994
Jersey[o]	1988	106	23 Aug 1994
Isle of Man[o]	1988	358	30 Jun 1994
Republic of Ireland[ox]	1989	91	1 Sep 1994
Sultanate of Oman[x]	1989	2	
Falkland Islands[x]	1989	1	
Switzerland[o]	1990	98	
France[o]	1990	9	
Denmark[x]	1992	1	
Portugal[ox]	1993	10	
Canada[x]	1993	1	
Germany[x]	1994	4	
Alderney[+]	1994	2	23 Aug 1994

o some or all cases in indigenous cattle
x exported from UK
+ exported from Guernsey

These are:

▲ the importation of BSE infected cattle directly or indirectly from a country with BSE

▲ the importation and use for feeding cattle with:

  a) infected compounded feed (*ie* containing MBM derived from infected ruminant animals from a country with scrapie and/or BSE)

  b) infected meat and bone meal or protein supplements as in a)

▲ the natural occurrence, in the country, of scrapie in sheep or goats at a significant level, in which the ratio of sheep to cattle was relatively high, and the waste offals were rendered to produce MBM for feeding, but under conditions that did not completely inactivate scrapie-like agents. This MBM would have to be incorporated at a significant inclusion rate in feed for young cattle destined for breeding and such cattle would need to be kept for at least 4 years. If sub-clinical BSE in cattle existed in a country this could also be a risk factor if similar conditions were met.

Whether BSE would be recognised if it occurred would depend on the ability of clinicians and pathologists to recognise and diagnose cases. This aspect has been dealt with by the issue of a video recording the clinical signs of BSE and by training experienced veterinary neuropathologists from the EU and round the world at three workshops held for the purpose at CVL. A full risk analysis by the United States Department of Agriculture (USDA) in the US indicated that there were few States in which BSE might occur. No cases have so far been found. A published risk assessment has also been performed in Argentina with the conclusions that BSE and scrapie are probably absent, unlikely to have been imported in the last 10 years and that it is virtually impossible for scrapie or BSE to enter the cattle population via feed. Some other countries, including Spain, have also conducted risk assessments with similar outcomes.

A few cases of BSE were the result of exporting from the UK, pre-clinically infected cattle to the Republic of Ireland, Sultanate of Oman, The Falkland Islands, Denmark, Portugal, Canada and Germany. However, it is now established that BSE has also occurred in indigenous cattle in the Republic of Ireland, Switzerland, Portugal and France (Table 2.2). Meat and bone meal seems to be incriminated in virtually every case where adequate records exist. Analysis shows that in one case in Switzerland MBM can be probably eliminated as a source of infection, though no alternative source has been identified. Whether the infected MBM was imported or derived only from waste tissues from indigenous scrapie-infected sheep is unknown, but the latter is most unlikely in Switzerland as there are relatively few sheep and goats compared to cattle, scrapie is extremely rare, and the rendering system (pressure cooking) is more likely to be consistently effective than in the UK.

No other country has the same degree of risk as the UK so that it can be expected that major epidemics of BSE are most unlikely elsewhere. Sporadic, low incidence BSE could occur where some of the important factors exist and controls are not in place (see above).

Suspect BSE cases that are negative for BSE

It is becoming more important, both for national and international studies, to study the 'BSE negative', *ie* unconfirmed, cases which form about 15% of the total suspected on clinical grounds in GB. The negative rate varies with the season of the year (higher in the spring when metabolic diseases are at a peak), is highest in very young and older cattle and lowest at the age (4-5 years) of peak incidence of BSE. Now that such cases are being studied at least one 'new' neurological condition has been recognised in old, predominantly beef, cows, mainly in Scotland (idiopathic brainstem neuronal necrosis and hippocampal sclerosis). This disease has epidemiological and pathological features that clearly distinguish it from BSE. Transmission studies are underway but no results are available yet. Negative cases are likely to be seen proportionately more frequently as the epidemic declines in the UK, and will need to be distinguished from atypical SEs. It will also be interesting to study the causes and incidence of these other diseases.

2.3 *New SEs of other species*

The studies of SEs of other species in the UK have also been important. Indeed disease was recognised in a captive wild ungulate, a nyala in a zoo, just before it was recognised in cattle (Table 1.2). As these species had been fed MBM for years before cases occurred it is likely that they, like cattle, were exposed after the rendering processes were altered. Further studies on greater kudu show that the incubation period is comparatively short, the incidence of disease is high, partly because there may be transmission from dam to offspring, and possibly horizontally too. Strain typing studies show that SE in the nyala and the first case in a greater kudu are associated with an agent that is indistinguishable from BSE. A much wider range of captive wild ungulates than the six species in which SE has been confirmed has been fed the same kind of feed, presumably with infection in it. This shows that there probably is a variation between species in susceptibility to the SE agent.

Until recently there was no evidence that FELIDAE (the cat family) were naturally affected by SEs even though their susceptibility to experimental infection with CJD has been known for years. However, since 1990 small numbers of feline SE (FSE) cases have been observed in domestic cats in the UK. The major pet food manufacturers voluntarily removed MBM and specified bovine and ovine offals from their products once the potential risks of infection of these tissues were recognised and before the SBO ban came into effect for humans in November 1989. However, it is likely that some animals were infected before these measures were taken. Though FSE in domestic cats is geographically widespread in Great Britain only 57 cases, out of an estimated population of over 7 million, have been reported between May 1990 and September 1994. No cats with confirmed disease were born after September 1990 when the SBO ban was extended to protect animals including cats from exposure.

The origin of the infection is presumed to be feed containing infected cattle offals but the precise origin in terms of a specific offal, or type of food (fresh, uncooked or cooked and processed) is not known. Meat and bone meal, as in cattle, could be a source. The varied diet of cats, especially over a lifetime, and the absence of historical feeding

records makes the epidemiological task of analysis a difficult one. At present, there are insufficient cases to secure a scientifically reliable result. One case of SE has been seen in a puma and four in cheetahs that had been fed uncooked cattle carcases unsuitable for human consumption (such as animals that had died or been killed on farm) containing central nervous tissue. Preliminary laboratory evidence indicates that isolates from three cases of SE in domestic cats behave in mice like BSE isolates. It is possible that the BSE agent is more pathogenic for these species than earlier strains of scrapie agent or that the exposure to BSE agent has been greater.

It has been suggested that there may be SEs of white tiger and ostrich, but the former has not been histologically confirmed and neither has been transmitted in the laboratory.

2.4 *The effectiveness of commercial rendering on the inactivation of scrapie and BSE agents*

Research of a very applied kind, and very difficult to design and execute, has been done on the effectiveness of some of the processes used in treating abattoir and butcher's waste to produce *inter alia* protein for consumption by animals. The difficulty arises because, in the case of the naturally occurring BSE agent a 1000-fold reduction in titre would be the maximum that could be detected. This may be insufficient to inspire the necessary confidence in decisions which are intended to rule out the presence of sufficient residual infectivity to cause disease. A large pool of BSE-infected cattle brains was prepared and mixed with abattoir waste (bones and alimentary tract) (see para 5.19). The mixture was then processed at temperatures and times representative of those used in various plants, using a pilot plant in which the process could be deliberately and accurately varied. The infectivity of the spike material and of the end-products are being measured by bioassay in mice and the loss of infectivity determined.

The results so far show that the spike titre is likely to be of the order of $10^{2.7}$ ID$_{50}$ mouse (i/c and i/p) infective units per gram. Residual infectivity has been detected after some of the low temperature/short time conditions of rendering. The experiment is complex and makes compromises in the selection of experimental processing methods. Also the low starting titre will not enable the true effectiveness of the more rigorous rendering systems to be fully established. The results do however, support the MBM hypothesis for the origin of the epidemic. A second experiment is also underway using an even larger pool of sheep brains from natural cases of scrapie in the UK. A third experiment using scrapie brains from other Member States has not started because of difficulties in collecting the necessary amount of tissue.

Even if a process is found which seems to eliminate a high proportion of infectivity it will still be difficult to decide whether it is safe to resume the use of MBM in cattle feeds. It is expected that, if all the controls are consistently applied and no significant routes of transmission other than feed exist, BSE will be eliminated. However, scrapie is likely to remain endemic in Britain, and scrapie agent may continue to be present in MBM. Furthermore, the Southwood Report, The Report of the Expert Group on Animal Feedingstuffs (Lamming Committee), and the SEAC consider the feeding of MBM to ruminants undesirable on general biological principles because ruminants are strict herbivores.

2.5 *Human transmissible spongiform encephalopathy*

CJD is the main TSE of man and has an almost worldwide incidence of about one case per two million per year. As there were fears that meat products from BSE-infected cattle, eaten before precautions were instituted in 1988 and 1989, might cause cases of CJD or a similar disease, it was decided to monitor human TSEs throughout the UK. The first results show that there has been no significant change in incidence since earlier decades but it is too early to draw any conclusions because the incubation period in kuru, for example, can exceed 30 years. There is also a similar study being conducted collaboratively in mainland Europe where BSE is reported to occur at a low incidence. Some other countries, such as Australia, will act as 'controls' since neither scrapie nor BSE exists there. The incidence of CJD in 1993 in four European countries (with and without BSE) was no different from that in the UK.

CJD cases occurring in human patients given human pituitary-derived growth hormone (hGH), show a different clinical pattern. Analysis of the nature of the clinical signs in all the human TSEs shows that in patients orally or peripherally exposed to kuru, hGH and human pituitary-derived gonadotrophin, the dominant presenting sign is ataxia whereas in sporadic CJD it is dementia. Therefore if BSE were transmitted to humans, it might be more likely to present with signs of ataxia than dementia and thus be distinguishable from sporadic CJD on clinical grounds. Occasional tragic cases of iatrogenic CJD from transplants and other surgical procedures continue to arise but fears that it might be transmitted by blood transfusion have not been supported by recent studies.

GSS continues to occur in a limited number of affected families. Fatal familial insomnia (FFI) has only been recognised recently. It is very rare, and although the association with an abnormal sequence of *PrP* gene is certain, the epidemiology is incomplete. It was suggested that there might be many cases other than typical CJD in which serious CNS disease, such as dementia, was associated with SE agents. However subsequent studies including a recent review of cases from which brain tissue was inoculated into animals in the USA, do not support this contention.

Reading list

ALPEROVITCH A, BROWN P, WEBER T, POCCHIARI M, HOFMAN A AND WILL R. (1994) Incidence of Creutzfeldt-Jakob disease in Europe in 1993. The Lancet *343*, 918.

BRADLEY R AND MATTHEWS D. (1992) Sub-acute, transmissible spongiform encephalopathies: current concepts and future needs. Rev. sci. tech. Off. int. Epiz. *11*, 605-634. (Lists countries reporting scrapie).

BRADLEY R AND WILESMITH J W. (1993) Epidemiology and control of bovine spongiform encephalopathy. Br. Med. Bull. *49*, 932-959.

BROWN P, GIBBS C J, RODGERS-JOHNSON P, ASHER D M, SULIMA M P, BACOTE A, GOLDFARB L G AND GAJDUSEK D C. (1994) Human spongiform encephalopathy - The National Institutes of Health series of 300 cases of experimentally transmitted disease. Ann. Neurol. *35*, 513-529.

DETWILER L A. (1992) Scrapie. Rev. sci. tech. Off. int. Epiz. *11*, 491-537.

FRASER H. (1991) Scrapie and its homologues. In*:* The Veterinary Annual (Thirty-first issue). Editors CSG Grunsell, Mary-Elizabeth Raw. Blackwell Scientific Publications, Oxford, pp 59-64.

HADLOW W J. (1991) To a better understanding of scrapie. In Sub-acute Spongiform Encephalopathies. Editors R Bradley, M Savey and B Marchant. Kluwer Academic Publishers, Dordrecht, pp 117-130.

HADLOW W J, KENNEDY R C, RACE R E AND EKLUND C M. (1980) Virologic and neurohistologic findings in dairy goats affected with natural scrapie. Vet. Pathol. *17*, 187-199.

HADLOW W J, KENNEDY R C AND RACE R E. (1982) Natural infection of suffolk sheep with scrapie virus. J. inf. Dis. *146*, 657-664.

KIMBERLIN R H. (1981) Scrapie. Br. vet. J. *137*, 105-112.

KIMBERLIN R H. (1986) Scrapie: how much do we really understand? Neuropathol appl. Neurobiol. *12*, 131-147.

KIMBERLIN R H. (1991) Scrapie. In: Diseases of Sheep (Second Edition). Editors W B Martin, I D Aitken. Blackwell Scientific Publications, Oxford, pp 163-169.

KIMBERLIN R H. (1992) Bovine spongiform encephalopathy. Rev. sci. tech. Off. int. Epiz. *11*, 347-390.

KIMBERLIN R H. (1993) Bovine spongiform encephalopathy. An appraisal of the current epidemic in the United Kingdom. Intervirology *35*, 208-218.

KIMBERLIN R H. (1994) A Scientific evaluation of research into bovine spongiform encephalopathy (BSE). In: Transmissible Spongiform Encephalopathies. Proceedings of a Consultation on BSE with the Scientific Veterinary Committee of the European Communities, held in Brussels, 14-15 September 1993. Editors R Bradley and B Marchant. CEC, Brussels, pp 455-477.

LIBERSKI PP. (1993) Subacute spongiform encephalopathies - the transmissible brain amyloidoses: a comparison with the non-transmissible brain amyloidoses of Alzheimer type. J. Comp. Path. *109*, 103-127.

PARRY H B. (1983) Scrapie disease in sheep. Historical, clinical epidemiological, pathological and practical aspects of the natural disease. Editor D R Oppenheimer. Academic Press, London, p 192.

PATTISON I H. (1972) Scrapie - a personal view. J. Clin. Path. 25 Suppl. (Roy. Coll. Path.) *6*, 110-114.

PATTISON I H. (1988) Fifty years with scrapie: a personal reminiscence. Vet. Rec. *123*, 661-666.

WILESMITH J W. (1991). The epidemiology of bovine spongiform encephalopathy. Semin. Virol. *2*, 239-245.

WILESMITH J W, RYAN J B M AND ATKINSON M J. (1991) Bovine spongiform encephalopathy: epidemiological studies on the origin. Vet. Rec. *128*, 199-203.

WILESMITH J W, RYAN J B M AND HUESTON W D. (1992) Bovine spongiform encephalopathy: case-control studies of calf feeding practices and meat and bone meal inclusion in proprietary concentrates. Res. Vet. Sci. *52*, 325-331.

WILESMITH J W, RYAN J B M, HUESTON W D AND HOINVILLE L J. (1992) Bovine spongiform encephalopathy: epidemiological features 1985 to 1990. Vet. Rec. *130*, 90-94.

WILESMITH J W, WELLS G A H, CRANWELL M P AND RYAN J B M. (1988) Bovine spongiform encephalopathy: epidemiological studies. Vet. Rec. *123*, 638-644.

CHAPTER

3

Genetics

3.1 *Introduction*

In several chapters of this report the importance of the host *PrP* gene, and in particular genetic variation, in all scrapie-like diseases has been made clear. For example, the pathogenesis (pattern of development of disease) including incubation period of experimental scrapie in mice and sheep is controlled by the interaction between the infectious agent (and its putative genome, which may be a nucleic acid), and at least one host gene: *Sinc/PrP* in mice and *Sip/PrP* in sheep. These genes were proposed to explain why different inbred lines of mice and sheep respectively, produced by selective breeding methods, responded to experimental challenge with unvarying strains of scrapie in consistent, but different ways. The incubation period of experimental BSE in mice may also be controlled by a second gene, or non-coding part of the *PrP* gene. This has been recognised because the incubation period of the experimental disease is different in two inbred mouse lines with the same *Sinc* genotype (s^7s^7) and also in two inbred lines with the same *Sinc* (p^7p^7) genotype.

3.2 *Molecular genetics*

Developments in molecular genetics have enabled a much greater understanding of scrapie-like diseases than hitherto. It is now possible to determine the *PrP* gene sequence in humans and animals by examination of the DNA extracted from a blood sample, or indeed any host tissue. In humans, relating variations in this sequence to the occurrence of any scrapie-like disease has enabled the identification of individuals at risk of

developing the diseases either, as some researchers hold, due to the *de novo* creation of the agent (*eg* in GSS and familial CJD), or as others hold, due to an increased susceptibility to disease caused by an infectious agent.

Familial disease

Disease that appears to run in families can be, but does not *have* to be, hereditary. If scrapie infection is present in a flock, rams and ewes of different *Sip* genotypes will show differing apparent susceptibility because of the influence of the genes on the incubation period, so that 'susceptible' and 'resistant' ewes may be bred by accident or design. In an infected but 'resistant' flock, the introduction of a ram with 'susceptibility' alleles will influence the occurrence of clinical scrapie in family lines in later generations thus giving the impression of a hereditary disease. There is also evidence that infectivity from the ewe can be transmitted via the placenta to offspring. This too will be observed as a familial type of transmission though it is more precisely called 'maternal' transmission. Maternal transmission includes both *in utero* and congenital infection, as well as that acquired in the immediate *post partum* period. Placental infection can also be transferred to unrelated sheep by contact or consumption *post partum,* and this is called horizontal or lateral transmission.

Human genetics

In humans sporadic, familial and acquired forms of CJD exist. Some researchers hold that post-translationally modified PrP^c (= PrP^{Sc}) certainly

Figure 3.1 Schematic representation of the 230 amino acid backbone of the human PrP protein showing sites of mutation associated with the occurrence of GSS at codons 102, 105, 117, 198 and 217

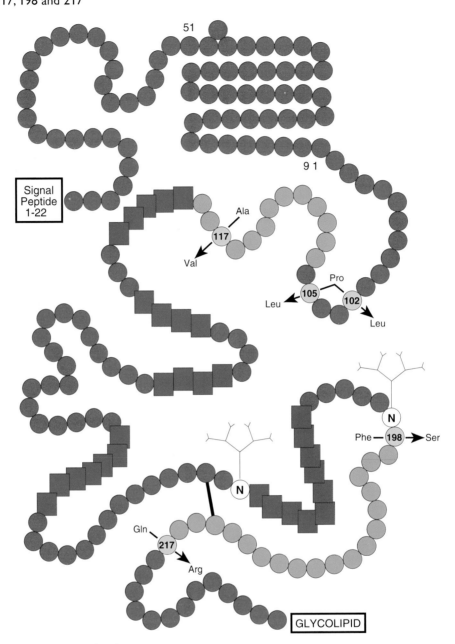

102 = proline-leucine
105 = proline-leucine
117 = alanine-valine
198 = phenylalanine-serine
217 = glutamine-arginine

The predicted secondary structure of PrP has a random turn and coil (magenta circles), α helix (orange circles), and β sheet configuration of amino acids (green rectangles). A disulphide bond links two cysteine residues at positions 179 and 214 and two complex sugar groups are attached to asparagine residues at positions 181 and 197. Other post-translational modifications involve cleavage of an N-terminus 22 residue signal peptide (top left) and replacement of a C-terminus 23 residue sequence by a glycophosphatidyl-inositol (GPI) membrane anchor labelled GLYCOLIPID. The octapeptide repeat region (top right) is shown with the normal five repeats.

Adapted from Brown P. (1994) The "Brave New World" of transmissible spongiform encephalopathy (infectious cerebral amyloidosis). Mol. Neurobiol. 8, 79-87, with permission.

plays a major role and may be entirely responsible for the disease. Identification of pathogenic mutations in the *PrP* gene (see para 1.24 and Figures 1.7 and 3.1) has enabled identification of some cases of apparently inherited prion disease that would have escaped diagnosis by means of conventional clinical and pathological criteria. At least one such case revealed no spongiform change in the brain. Some have claimed an abundance of such cases but this has been refuted. However, identification of a mutation which is pathogenic only in later life is insufficient evidence by which to confirm the diagnostic neurological illness unless supported by additional pathology. *PrP* gene mutations do not invariably lead to disease even in patients who live long enough to enter the at-risk age class. For example, only about 50% of patients with the codon 200 mutation die of the disease. In genetic terms the penetrance is 50% and the risk of developing disease in a full lifespan, 1 in 2. New mutations are continually being discovered.

There is considerable overlap in the clinical and pathological features of human neurodegenerative disorders so the new tools of molecular genetics are contributing significantly to the differential diagnosis and epidemiology of these diseases. It has to be remembered however, that CJD of man is rare, and that the familial sub-groups form only about 15% of the total and the iatrogenic sub-group even less. Nevertheless, with advances in genetic knowledge, techniques and counselling, improved management of the familial forms of the human disease should be possible in the future. Preventative medicine also may have a role to play in the future as chemical or genetic methods for delaying or preventing disease progression are developed. However, it will also be important to deal with the formidable ethical problems that this will raise for all those involved.

Genetic variation

That genes, and particularly the *PrP* gene, are important in TSEs is indisputable. However, there seems to be more variation in the gene in some species than in others and research has to be done to decide which variations have effects on the pathogenesis of the diseases.

Sheep genetics

In sheep scrapie the incubation period-controlling *Sip* gene (the ovine equivalent of *Sinc* in mice) has two alleles sA and pA. These alleles segregate with short and prolonged incubation period respectively with at least some scrapie strains (next para and para 5.2) in some breeds of sheep. *PrP* gene polymorphisms are associated with both alleles of *Sip* and with the occurrence of natural scrapie in several sheep breeds. In this context, NPU Cheviot sheep homozygous for the sA allele are more likely to succumb to scrapie following experimental challenge with SSBP I ('A' group) scrapie (see paras 1.8 and 3.7) than pApA sheep. The animals are not completely resistant or susceptible as apparent resistance can sometimes be overcome by more challenging routes of exposure. Not all breeds of sheep show the common polymorphism at codon 136 associated with susceptibility, but nevertheless some have different responses to natural scrapie exposure. There is still much to be learned about the role of other polymorphisms of the *PrP* gene, and perhaps other genes, in sheep scrapie. As more molecular genetic investigations are reported, so the subject becomes clearer. The main problem is that there are more alleles of the ovine *PrP* gene than of the *Sip* gene, though fewer than there are in the human *PrP* gene, so the subject of *PrP* genotype and occurrence of familial CJD in humans is more complex. A further complication is that there is a variable interaction with different scrapie agent strains.

Interaction of *Sip* and agent strain groups in sheep

It is important to note the differences in outcome following experimental challenge of sheep of differing *Sip* genotype with the CH1641 isolate of scrapie. This is the single member of the 'C' group of scrapie isolates. In contrast to all the other 'A' group isolates of scrapie, the alleles of *Sip* operate in the opposite direction, with the incubation period being shorter in pApA homozygotes than in sAsA homozygotes, but incidences (resistance and susceptibility) are much the same. If such a strain were prevalent in the national sheep population and one bred for 'resistance' by selecting for pApA genotype, then the results could prove to be disastrous if selected 'resistant' sheep and a C type agent strain were to come into contact. (Note: only 'A' and 'C' strains have been categorised. There is no Group 'B' strain).

BSE agent operates in the same way as the CH1641 scrapie strain in Cheviot sheep in the NPU flock. That is to say that, at least in the pApA sheep, there is a relatively short incubation period and incomplete incidence of disease suggesting the segregation of other alleles of *Sip* and variants of the *PrP* gene in this flock. However, BSE agent is not CH1641. This is easily established because BSE readily transmits to all four inbred strains of experimental mice whereas CH1641 does not. In the NPU Cheviot sheep flock the response to challenge with 'A' group (SSBP I) strains of scrapie (*ie* those that have short and long incubation periods in *Sip* sAsA and pApA sheep respectively) is completely explained by *PrP* gene variation at codon 136 which coincides with the alleles of *Sip*. By contrast the response of sheep to the 'C' group strains (CH1641 and BSE *ie* those that have long and short incubation periods in *Sip* sAsA and pApA sheep respectively) is associated with allelic variation at codon 171. These issues are described in detail in the publications of Goldmann *et al* 1994 and Hunter *et al* 1993 which are in the reading list.

Cattle genetics

By contrast, in cattle, three polymorphisms have been found in the *PrP* gene. Two are silent (not resulting in an amino acid change) whereas the third occurs as either five or six copies of the octapeptide repeat sequence thus giving opportunity for 5/5, 6/5 or 6/6 genotypes. None of the three polymorphisms appears to be related to BSE occurrence. However, it is of interest that the 5/5 genotype is rare in Holstein Friesian cattle though it occurs more frequently in other breeds such as the Guernsey.

Experimental BSE develops preferentially (*ie* with shortest periods of incubation) in mice and sheep of certain *PrP* genotypes. However, cattle seem, as far as has been determined at present, to be uniformly susceptible to natural and experimental BSE. They thus behave like goats and Syrian hamsters which seem to be uniformly susceptible to experimental

scrapie, and mink which are similarly universally susceptible to TME. Reasons that explain these species/agent differences remain to be discovered.

PrP gene in captive wild ruminants and other species

PrP gene sequences have been analysed in Arabian oryx and greater kudu. The oryx gene had only one amino acid difference in the encoded protein from that of the sheep. The greater kudu *PrP* gene differed from the sheep and the bovine genes by 7 and 5 amino acids respectively. Four of these amino acid differences from the bovine gene are common to sheep and kudu. The *PrP* gene sequence has been established in the hamster, mink and pig and partial sequence data are available for the marmoset. More work needs to be done to evaluate the biological significance of these findings in relation to species barriers and to collect similar data from cats and other species or individuals susceptible or apparently resistant to BSE and other TSE agents.

3.3 *Population genetics*

A conventional pedigree analysis has been conducted in home-bred pedigree Holstein Friesian herds in which at least one case of BSE has been confirmed. The study did not indicate the possibility of horizontal or vertical transmission but did show a substantial familial aggregation of animals with disease. However, separation of the genetic and environmental factors that may contribute to disease occurrence has not been possible. The segregation ratios in progeny of parents identified as potential carriers of the 'susceptibility allele', on the assumption of a recessive model of inheritance, do not contradict the hypothesis of a recessive model with complete penetrance. (Note: a recessive model implies that the gene responsible would only have a phenotypic effect if present in the homozygous state *ie* that both alleles were the same). Nevertheless, the fit of the model is confounded by the absence of disease in offspring of considerable age where both parents were affected, and by the less than 50% incidence in offspring derived from affected cows mated to putative carrier bulls.

The authors claim that the evidence to date shows that genetic models fit the pattern of disease better than non-genetic models and that a recessive form of inheritance is more likely than a dominant one. There are remaining puzzles however. For example, why did all the randomly selected, parenterally-challenged cattle succumb to BSE after a similar incubation period, and why is there a lack of a clear sire effect? Current results of the statistical modelling of the genetics do not indicate that susceptibility to BSE has a major genetic component.

Reading list

COLLINGE J AND PALMER S. (1993) Prion diseases in humans and their relevance to other neurodegenerative diseases. Dementia *4*, 178-185.

CURNOW R N, WIJERATNE W V S AND HAU C M. (1994) The inheritance of susceptibility to BSE. In: Transmissible Spongiform Encephalopathies. Proceedings of a Consultation on BSE with the Scientific Veterinary Committee of the Commission of the European Communities, held in Brussels, 14-15 September 1993. Editors R Bradley and B Marchant. CEC, Brussels, pp 109-124.

ETHICAL PROBLEMS IN GENETIC COUNSELLING. (1993) Bioethics, Nuffield Foundation, .

FOSTER J D AND DICKINSON A G. (1988) The unusual properties of CH1641, a sheep-passaged isolate of scrapie. Vet. Rec. *123*, 5-8.

FOSTER J D, HOPE J AND FRASER J. (1993) Transmission of bovine spongiform encephalopathy to sheep and goats. Vet. Rec. *133*, 339-341.

GOLDFARB L G, BROWN P AND GAJDUSEK D C. (1992) The molecular genetics of human transmissible spongiform encephalopathy. In: Prion Diseases of Humans and Animals. Editors S B Prusiner, J Collinge, J Powell and B Anderton. Ellis Horwood,Chichester, pp 139-153.

GOLDMANN W, HUNTER N, BENSON G, FOSTER J D AND HOPE J. (1991) Different scrapie-associated fibril proteins (PrP) are encoded by lines of sheep selected for different alleles of the *Sip* gene. J. Gen. Virol. *72*, 2411-2417.

GOLDMANN W, HUNTER N, SMITH G, FOSTER J AND HOPE J. (1994) PrP genotype and agent effects in scrapie: change in allelic interaction with different isolates of agent in sheep, a natural host of scrapie. J. Gen. Virol. *75*, 989-995.

HUNTER N, FOSTER J D AND HOPE J. (1992) Natural scrapie in British sheep: breeds, ages and PrP gene polymorphisms. Vet. Rec. *130*, 389-392.

HUNTER N, GOLDMANN W, BENSON G, FOSTER J D AND HOPE J. (1994) *PrP* genotype studies. In: Transmissible Spongiform Encephalopathies. Proceedings of a Consultation on BSE with the Scientific Veterinary Committee of the Commission of the European Communities, held in Brussels, 14-15 September 1993. Editors R Bradley and B Marchant. CEC, Brussels, pp 125-139.

HUNTER N AND HOPE J. (1991) The genetics of scrapie susceptibility in sheep (and its implications for BSE). In: Breeding for Disease Resistance in Farm Animals. Editors J B Owen and RFE Axford. CAB International, Wallingford, pp 329-344.

PALMER M S AND COLLINGE J. (1993) Mutations and polymorphisms in the prion protein gene. Human Mutation *2*, 168-173.

POIDINGER M, KIRKWOOD J AND ALMOND J W. (1993) Sequence analysis of the PrP protein from two species of antelope susceptible to transmissible spongiform encephalopathy. Arch. Virol. *131*, 193-199.

CHAPTER 4

Pathogenesis and Pathology

4.1 *Tissue assays and titrations*

Once a susceptible experimental host is identified one can quantify the amount of infectivity present in the brain or other tissues. Tissue is usually homogenized in 10 volumes of saline and inoculated into the brain of mice (i/c). Liquids such as serum or cerebrospinal fluid can be inoculated undiluted. Titrations are done by making serial dilutions to give 1/100, 1/1000, 1/10,000 dilutions and so on. Equal volumes of these dilutions are inoculated i/c into groups of mice. Mice are then observed clinically for signs of disease which is confirmed by microscopic examination of the brain. If no disease results in the lifespan of the mouse there is no detectable infectivity in the inoculum. The amount of infectivity in the sample can be calculated from the number of animals dying after receiving each dilution. The dilution at which 50% of the mice are killed (ID_{50}) is the end point and the number of ID_{50} (the titre) per gram of the source material can be calculated. Different tissues give different titres depending on the mode of pathogenesis and the stage in the incubation period or of clinical disease when the donor is killed or dies. It is also possible to construct a curve relating incubation period to the dose given, but this is different with different strains of animals and agent.

Once the bioassay for infectivity was developed it was possible to detect and titrate the amount of infectious agent in the tissues of cases of TSEs and in experimental models of these conditions. It was established in the 1960s and 1970s that in scrapie the highest concentrations were to be found in the brain and spinal cord of a clinically, terminally affected animal; however smaller amounts were

found in the spleen and other elements of the lymphoreticular system (LRS), and occasionally in other tissues. Systematic studies showed that during the incubation period there was a zero phase in some models during which infectivity could not be detected; it then appeared in the spleen and related organs and later in the CNS as shown in Figure 1.1. This general pattern was seen in pioneering studies done in mice in the UK. The model showed clearly that, following infection, replication of the agent occurred in the lymphoreticular system, and this was an essential prelude to the invasion and replication in the CNS.

4.2 *Sinc gene*

In mice the *Sinc* gene is a major determinant of the incubation period, interacting closely with the strain of the agent. The long incubation period and slow progress of scrapie is due to restrictions on the process of replication in different tissues. This is due to the availability of only a finite number of replication sites in a restricted number of non-replaceable cells. The interaction between strain of agent and *Sinc* controls intracellular replication and/or the transcellular spread of infection in at least two stages of pathogenesis: first at the LRS/nervous tissue interface, probably on the latter side because the effects of *Sinc* are less obvious in the LRS. The second stage is within the peripheral and central nervous systems (CNS) and also involves the targeting of infection to specific CNS areas. However, the expression of the *Sinc/PrP* gene in the LRS is also important because mice from which the gene has been deleted seem to be totally resistant to experimental infection. In mice the scrapie agent replicates to produce a moderate titre in the LRS tissues (notably spleen) but then levels off. Some time after infection of the LRS, infectivity passes, probably via the splanchnic nerve, to the thoracic cord and then passes caudally and rostrally to infect the brainstem and subsequently the fore brain. Further replication of the agent in the CNS finally produces higher titres than in the LRS tissues. Some mouse models permit infection and replication in the LRS but no neuroinvasion or disease occurs during the lifespan of the animal. It seems likely that the same principles of agent strain and host genotype (*PrP* gene) interactions apply in other TSEs. Other genes may also control the incubation period in mice of different inbred strains. This is because when different mouse strains with the same *Sinc* genotypes are challenged intracerebrally with BSE agent, incubation periods of differing length are observed.

4.3   *Pathogenesis of natural scrapie*

In goats and Suffolk sheep with natural clinical scrapie, the distribution of infectivity within the tissues is consistent with that found in mice experimentally challenged with certain strains of murine scrapie. Furthermore, studies of the infectivity of tissues during the incubation period of natural scrapie in Suffolk sheep show that infection is detectable in the LRS before the CNS. This does not prove that pathogenesis is the same in sheep and mice but it makes an acceptable hypothesis. Other evidence points to infectivity of the placenta and thus the opportunity for maternal transmission. This does not occur in experimental rodent models of scrapie and some of the other diseases. Since the nasal mucosa of sheep with natural scrapie contains infectivity this raises the possibility of transmission between sheep via nasal secretions. The consistent finding of infectivity in the LRS of the gut strongly points to alimentary exposure, but not necessarily to alimentary excretion since scrapie agent has not been found in faeces even of clinically affected animals. In breeds other than Suffolks, the same general pattern is seen in the distribution of agent but titres are often lower, probably because of differences in the efficiency of the bioassays of different strains of agent in mice.

4.4   *Pathogenesis in experimental BSE and natural TME*

The pathogenesis of BSE is in the process of being determined, but there is no reason to believe that it is fundamentally different from that in other TSEs. The fact that in terminal clinical cases of BSE, infectivity has been found only in the CNS does not exclude a role for the LRS in pathogenesis because studies of scrapie in mice show that the process of neuroinvasion can be initiated when infectivity titres in the LRS are low. Indeed, preliminary results in 1994 (see below and para 5.13) have shown that following experimental oral challenge of calves with large doses (100g) of brain from confirmed BSE cases, though no clinical disease has resulted in those animals still alive at 32 months of age, there was evidence for infectivity of the distal ileum (which contains Peyer's patches which are composed of LRS tissue) in calves killed at 10 months and 14 months of age, 6 and 10 months after dosing. This experiment is incomplete. It should also be remembered that bioassays of BSE agent infectivity are conducted in mice (as were those of scrapie agent from natural cases of scrapie in goats and Suffolk sheep), across a species barrier, which is likely to reduce sensitivity. The situation with BSE may resemble that in TME. In the latter disease, bioassays can be performed within species, that is, in mink. Pathogenesis studies of experimental TME showed only small amounts of infectivity in extra-neural tissues, which may be the reason colony mink are not natural hosts for the agent.

The large pathogenesis experiment in cattle experimentally challenged with BSE brain referred to above and described in more detail in para 5.13 should reveal the time during the incubation period when neuro-invasion of the CNS can be detected and the sequential infectivity titres in different CNS locations. It may also determine whether or not any detectable infectivity occurs in other parts of the LRS than distal ileum during incubation, and if so, from which tissues it is eliminated by the time clinical signs become apparent. Because the bioassay of infectivity is across a species barrier (from cattle to mice) a limited number of assays of brain, spleen and lymph nodes are being done concurrently in mice and cattle and the ratio of titres in the brain in the two species will indicate whether, and to what extent, the titres are underestimated in mice.

4.5 *PrP^Sc accumulation and cellular changes*

Recent work has focused on the nature of the spongiform changes and their distribution within the CNS. Immunological staining of brain tissue from cases of experimental murine scrapie examined by electron microscopy, shows that *in vivo,* PrP^Sc accumulates outside cells before and during the appearance of the typical cytoplasmic vacuoles. This may be because, being partially protease resistant, it is not catabolised as the normal form is. *In vitro,* PrP^Sc is located within cells in the lysosomal organelle system. *In vitro,* the vacuoles, when they appear, also stain for lysosomal markers

and for ubiquitin (a heat shock protein) and normal Tau proteins, these being common elements of neuronal degeneration. It has been suggested that those changes are the result of a disorder of membrane function caused by the accumulated PrP^Sc (Figure 4.1). PrP^Sc also polymerises to form amyloid plaques. Using intraocular challenge of the mouse it has been possible to define how infectivity placed in the eye moves along the optic tracts to produce pathological changes in the contralateral colliculi* or lateral geniculate nucleus* (depending on the strain of agent and mouse *Sinc* genotype).

_____

* Note: These are anatomical parts of the brain concerned with processing information from the retina (eye).

Figure 4.1 The sites of PrP^C formation (processing and trafficking) from endoplasmic reticulum (ER) through the Golgi etc to the plasma membrane etc, where PrP^Sc is formed as shown by the heavy arrows. *In vivo* PrP^Sc is deposited also in both intracellular spaces and extracellular spaces, sometimes in the form of amyloid PrP^Sc -positive plaques

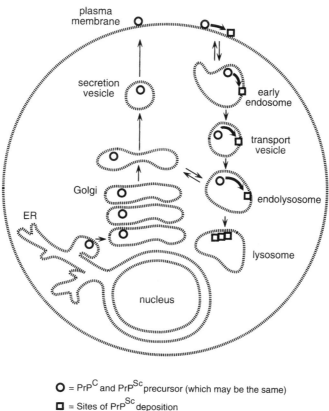

O = PrP^C and PrP^Sc precursor (which may be the same)
□ = Sites of PrP^Sc deposition

Adapted from Caughey B, Race R and Chesebro B (1992) Effects of scrapie infection on cellular PrP metabolism. In: Prion Diseases of Humans and Animals. S B Prusiner, J Collinge, J Powell and B Anderton, eds. Ellis Horwood, Chichester, pp 445-456.

4.6 *Neurohistopathology and PrP^{Sc} detection*

From the practical point of view it has been found that BSE, like scrapie, can be effectively diagnosed and distinguished from other types of neurological disease by neuropathological examination of selected areas of the CNS. The lesions consist of spongiform change in grey matter neuropil (Figure

Table 4.1 Similiar behaviour in mice of isolates of BSE, FSE and SE agents recovered from other species - and differences from scrapie

| | Mouse strain or cross | | | | |
| | *Sinc^{s7}* | | *Sinc^{p7}* | | *Sinc^{s7p7}* |
Source	RIII	C57BL	VM	IM	C57BL×VM
BSE:					
cow 1	328±3	438±7	471±8	537±7	not tested
cow 2	327±4	407±4	499±8	548±9	743±14
cow 3	316±3	436±6	518±7	561±9	not tested
cow 4	314±3	423±5	514±11	565±8	not tested
cow 5	321±4	444±14	516±9	577±12	745±22
cow 6	319±3	447±11	545±7	576±13	755±18
cow 7	335±7	475±14	545±12	not tested	unfinished
Scrapie:					
sheep 1	386±10	404±5	769±16	815±23	610±8
sheep 2	-ve	-ve	-ve	-ve	-ve
sheep 3	612±28	618±27	-ve	unfinished	unfinished
FSE:					
cat 1[a]	348±3	434±12	542±12	573±13	731±23
cat 2	312±4	426±4	457±10	523±10	676±13
cat 3	302±3	405±8	469±12	502±14	692±10
SE:					
kudu[a]	339±5	465±14	536±10	560±12	754±24
nyala[a]	378±8	529±11	548±17	614±11	772±3
Experimental BSE:					
sheep	297±3	408±9	446±10	478±9	662±13
goat	308±3	392±8	480±11	512±12	685±14
pig	316±5	433±6	489±8	534±16	717±11

[a] Transmission from formol-fixed tissue

Mean incubation periods (days ± SEM) in transmissions of spongiform encephalopathies to mice

Note also the uniform response of isolate from most species and the variable responses to different isolates of scrapie.

From Bruce M, Chree A, McConnell I, Foster J, Pearson G and Fraser H. (1994) Transmission of bovine spongiform encephalopathy and scrapie to mice: strain variation and the species barrier. Phil. Trans. Roy. B. *343*, 405-411.

1.4A), neuronal loss, neuronal vacuolation (Figure 1.4B), astrogliosis, and more rarely development of amyloid plaques. Diagnosis can be supplemented by detection of PrPSc in the form of fibrils (SAF-scrapie associated fibrils) in extracts of brain tissue examined by electron microscopy (Figure 1.6) or immunologically by immunoblotting (Figures 1.5A and 1.5B), or by immunocytochemistry of tissue sections. This last mentioned technique shows that significant accumulation of PrP consistently occurs in association with spongiform change.

4.7 Strain typing

Strain typing is done by intracerebral inoculation and passage in four inbred strains of mice of a homozygous *Sinc* genotype, and one F1 hybrid, and observing the length of the incubation period and lesion profile. The severity and distribution of the brain lesions provide a means of typing isolates and laboratory strains of SE agents which is independent of the method of strain typing based on the measurement of incubation period in inbred mice of different *Sinc/PrP* genotypes. The type of lesion in the CNS may also vary with the strain of agent, for example, the occurrence of PrPSc-positive, congophilic, amyloid plaques or white matter vacuolation.

Strain typing studies of BSE have produced a number of findings with important implications. For instance it has been shown that the BSE isolates so far studied, from cases occurring in different parts of the UK, and in different years, are indistinguishable from each other, but distinct from all previously studied laboratory strains of scrapie.

Recent transmissions to mice of spongiform encephalopathy from five animals of three species naturally infected with SE (3 cats, 1 greater kudu, 1 nyala) and one animal of each of three species experimentally infected with BSE (sheep, goat, pig), have given similar results to those resulting from transmission from cattle naturally affected with BSE (Table 4.1). Thus in each case the agent causing disease in mice is presumably the BSE agent which has retained its identity when naturally or experimentally passaged through a range of species of different *PrP* gene sequences. According to the prion hypothesis however, the donor species

should contribute chemically different PrP to the agent. Hence, the donor species is with respect to BSE a source of very little variation of the disease characteristics in mice. This argues for the presence of an agent-specific informational molecule additional to PrP *ie* for the presence of a specific agent genome.

When BSE or scrapie are transmitted from the natural host to mice the incubation periods are usually long compared with subsequent mouse to mouse passages due to the donor species effect (see para 1.12, Figure 1.2 and paras 5.5 and 5.6). Contributory factors to this effect are the relatively low efficiency of trans-species transmission, the selection of mutant strains which more readily replicate in the new species, and a modification of pathogenesis (this can include a failure of intracerebrally-inoculated infection to establish itself directly in the brain which is why mice were injected by both i/c and i/p routes).

4.8 Pathogenesis of CNS disease

Little is known about the nervous malfunction that gives rise to the typical clinical picture of the various TSEs. Widespread neuronal degeneration and loss probably explains the dementia, but it is not clear what causes the recently described abnormalities of rumination in BSE, or the characteristic EEG of CJD. It seems likely however, that clinical disease is associated with agent replication, accumulation of PrPSc and consequent cell dysfunction in specific clinical target areas. An impressive feature of natural and experimental BSE in cattle is the uniform distribution of vacuolar lesions in the CNS. Thus given the apparent singularity of the BSE agent associated with the epidemic and the uniform susceptibility of cattle to experimental infection, it seems that infection of the CNS commences at a specific site in the spinal cord which determines the neural pathways by which infection spreads to the clinical target areas.

It may be that other biochemical changes may be found that are associated with the pathology of TSE. Nuclear magnetic resonance (NMR) studies of scrapie-affected mice show an abnormal signal in brain, and electrochemical analysis of urine from BSE and scrapie-affected cattle and sheep has also indicated abnormalities. The molecular bases of these findings have yet to be discovered but they may provide usable diagnostic tests, at least for problem cases.

The consistency of the pathology of natural and experimental BSE in cattle strongly supports the evidence that only one major strain of agent is responsible. In contrast, the 'lesion profile' in sheep with scrapie is much more varied. The lesion profiles in cats and captive wild ruminants differ from BSE in cattle, presumably because of their differing *PrP* gene sequences. For example, the pathology in domestic and wild FELIDAE is much more florid than in BSE of cattle and lesions are prominent in the cerebrum and thalamus. But the lesions produced by the isolates in mice from domestic cats, the nyala and greater kudu seem indistinguishable, strongly supporting the view that only one strain of agent is involved in all the new TSEs identified since 1986.

Reading list

BRUCE, M, CHREE A, McCONNELL I, FOSTER J, PEARSON G AND FRASER H. (1994) Transmission of bovine spongiform encephalopathy and scrapie to mice: strain variation and the species barrier. Phil. Trans. Roy. Soc. B *343*, 405-411.

BÜELER H, AGUZZI A, SAILER A, GREINER R A, AUTENRIED P, AGUET M AND WEISSMANN C. (1993) Mice devoid of PrP are resistant to scrapie. Cell *73*, 1339-1347.

CZUB M, BRAIG H R AND DIRINGER H. (1986) Pathogenesis of scrapie: Study of the temporal development of clinical symptoms of infectivity titres and scrapie-associated fibrils in brains of hamsters infected intraperitoneally. J. Gen. Virol. *67*, 2005-2009.

EKLUND C M, KENNEDY R C AND HADLOW W J. (1967) Pathogenesis of scrapie virus infection in the mouse. J. Inf. Dis. *117*, 15-22.

FRASER H AND DICKINSON A G. (1968) The sequential development of the brain lesions of scrapie in three strains of mice. J. Comp. Path. *78*, 301-311.

HADLOW W J, KENNEDY R C AND RACE R E. (1982) Natural infection of Suffolk sheep with scrapie virus. J. Inf. Dis. *146*, 657-664.

HADLOW W J, RACE R E AND KENNEDY R C. (1987) Temporal distribution of transmissible mink encephalopathy virus in mink inoculated subcutaneously. J. Virol. *61*, 3235-3240.

JEFFREY M, GOODSIR C M, BRUCE M E, McBRIDE P A, SCOTT J R AND HALLIDAY W G. (1992) Infection specific prion protein (PrP) accumulates on neuronal plasmalemma in scrapie infected mice. Neurosci. Lett. *147*, 106-109.

KIMBERLIN R H. (1990) Unconventional "slow" viruses. In: Topley and Wilson's Principles of Bacteriology, Virology and Immunity. 8th Edition. L H Collier and M C Timbury, Eds. Edward Arnold, London, *4*, 671-693.

KIMBERLIN R H AND WALKER C A. (1988) Incubation periods in six models of intraperitoneally injected scrapie depend mainly on the dynamics of agent replication within the nervous system and not the lymphoreticular system. J. Gen. Virol. *69*, 2953-2960.

KIMBERLIN R H AND WALKER C A. (1988) Pathogenesis of experimental scrapie. In: Novel Infectious Agents and the Central Nervous System. Ciba Foundation Symposium No. 135. G. Bock and J Marsh, Eds. Wiley, Chichester, pp 37-62.

KIMBERLIN R H AND WALKER C A. (1989) Pathogenesis of scrapie in mice after intragastric infection. Virus Res. *12*, 213-220.

SCOTT J R AND FRASER H. (1989) Enucleation after intraocular scrapie injection delays the spread of infection. Brain Res. *504*, 301-305.

WELLS G A H AND McGILL I S. (1992) Recently described scrapie-like encephalopathies of animals: case definitions. Res. Vet. Sci. *53*, 1-10.

Transmission

5.1 *Introduction*

Transmission is an all embracing word encompassing natural transmission and experimental transmission from one animal to another of the same or different species. Brain is often used as the source material as it usually has the highest titre and is least contaminated by other pathogens when expertly collected. Transmission studies reveal the experimental host range for a particular agent or agent strain causing, or associated with, the primary case and the presence and amount of infectivity in other tissues. The amount of infectivity (its titre) is determined by inoculation of increasing dilutions of tissue until an end point is reached (see para 4.1). The information gained from these studies can assist in the assessment of possible risks for susceptible species or animal groups.

Transmissibility is the fundamental criterion for establishing membership of the TSE group of diseases and also is of great practical value in devising methods for their control. For example, if a new natural TSE is confirmed in a food animal species, safety administrators will wish to know the pathogenesis, tissue distribution of agent and its concentration in order to develop safety guidelines and regulations to protect animal and public health. The same applies if disease occurs in a species donating tissues or body fluids for use in surgery or preparing biological products.

The only available method to assess the hazards and risks is the use of animal bioassays. It is most convenient to use experimental rodents where suitable models are available. However not all

diseases transmit directly to rodents. Neither is transmission guaranteed at every attempt. For example, CJD from Caucasian patients in the USA is more readily transmissible to primates than mice whereas CJD in Japanese patients transmits to rats and mice in some 80% of attempts. Even with scrapie not all isolates transmit to mice, the most commonly used laboratory animal. BSE however, has been transmitted by parenteral inoculation to mice from brain material of affected animals on every occasion it has been attempted, though the number of transmissions is small.

Tissue culture systems exist but cannot yet be used for detecting infectivity as they are insufficiently sensitive and may not support or replicate all field strains. Lines of mice transgenic for *PrP* genes of other species are being studied but it is too early to say if these will be helpful to assess the risks from particular agents to these species. It is obvious that any test for the agent which was simpler and quicker than mouse inoculation could have markedly improved the speed and precision of monitoring and controlling the BSE epidemic. Development of such a test must continue to be a target of molecular studies.

5.2 *Agent strains*

Though in BSE it appears that only one strain of agent is responsible for the epidemic, and this is one reason why the clinical signs and lesion profile in cattle show very little variation, the situation in sheep scrapie is probably different. There is a degree of variation in clinical signs, and even more variation in the lesion profile in brains of sheep with natural scrapie that suggests there may be different strains of scrapie agent in the national flock, though some of this variation could be due to variation in *PrP* genotype. About 20 different laboratory strains of scrapie agent have been identified by the characteristics of the incubation period and lesion profile in certain inbred strains of mice. This is a difficult and tedious method but nevertheless provides unique and valuable information. The mice must be of very high health status in order to survive the long incubation period. Their genetic status (both *Sinc* genotype and genetic background) must be known and maintained constant in order to give consistent and interpretable results.

Furthermore, rigorous laboratory procedures must be used to avoid cross-contamination. Thus only a limited number of such tests can be done and need to be conducted in specialist laboratories. Account must also be taken of the *Sinc* genotype as well as differences in breeding lines with the same *Sinc* genotype which can (after challenge with BSE agent, for example) respond differently to the same isolate.

5.3   *Efficiency of different routes of infection*

Routes of infection considerably affect the infectious dose (ID) of agent required to produce disease. Parenteral exposure is more certain to produce disease than alimentary (oral) exposure. Intracerebral challenge is more likely to be effective than intravenous, which in turn is likely to be more effective than intra-peritoneal or sub-cutaneous challenge. For example, in mice challenged with the 139A strain of scrapie, the effective exposure by the intragastric route was about 5 $\log^{10}$ units (100,000 fold) less efficient than with the intracerebral route, *ie* 1 intragastric ID = 10^5 intracerebral ID. These differences in efficiency of the oral route are found within a species, but recent experiments have enabled similar estimations to be made between cattle and mice, *ie* across a species barrier. The effective difference in transmission efficiency by the intracerebral and oral routes was also about 5 orders of magnitude. Experimental challenge of mice by the conjunctival route gives incubation periods comparable with some other peripheral routes of challenge.

5.4   *Effective exposure*

The transmission of TSE infection from one species to another depends on the 'effective exposure'. This in turn depends upon three factors; the dose, the route of exposure and the extent of the species barrier (see para 5.5). The dose depends on the mass or volume of the material given and its infectivity titre.

5.5   *The species barrier*

When transmission between species does occur, the incubation period at second and subsequent passage within the recipient species is shorter, dose for dose and for the same route of challenge, than the primary passage across the species barrier. The species barrier has two components: the strain of agent, and the donor species effect which seems to be determined (at least in part) by the *PrP* gene sequence of the donor and recipient species. In some species, *eg* sheep and mice, there can also be a 'barrier' to the transmission of the same strain of scrapie within species. This barrier is determined by the *Sip* and *Sinc* gene sequences respectively (and presumptively by the *PrP* gene which is probably the same gene). Whether it is ever genuinely impossible to cross species boundaries is an untested hypothesis.

5.6   *Donor species effect*

When there is no change in the strain of agent on crossing the species barrier, the difference in incubation period between the first passage in the new species compared to the second is due to the 'donor species effect'. This component of the species barrier probably has to do with the difference in the nucleotide sequence of the *PrP* gene of the donor and recipient species. Where the homology is close, transmission may be more likely than where the differences are large, depending on the agent strain. The 'donor species effect' may be due to the donor PrP^{Sc} being different from the recipient PrP^{C} but only if PrP^{Sc} is a component of the agent; otherwise it is another protein that is important. Thus the most sensitive system for determining the infectivity of tissues is usually to use intracerebral inoculations in the same species.

In practice such systems may be prohibitively expensive and of course are impossible for agents isolated from human cases.

5.7 *Natural host range of TSE agents*

An attempt is made in the following paragraphs to summarise what we know of the transmissibility of certain diseases to specific hosts.

5.8 *Transmission from man to man*

Kuru

Kuru was probably transmitted by a combination of consumption, ocular exposure and skin (wound) exposure to the infected, uncooked and cooked tissues of dead patients at mortuary rituals of the Fore people of the eastern highlands in Papua New Guinea. The number of cases has greatly decreased after cannibalism ceased in the late 1950s though a small number of incidents still occur with an incubation period of over 30 years.

Iatrogenic CJD

CJD has occurred in a few patients following exposure to instruments or materials derived from infected human tissues. These were:-

▲ implanted brain electrodes

▲ neurosurgical instruments

▲ corneal graft

▲ dura mater grafts

▲ human pituitary-derived growth hormone

▲ human pituitary-derived gonadotrophin

The use of hormones extracted from human cadaveric pituitaries for use in humans has now been suspended in the UK.

5.9 *Transmission from animals to animals*

Iatrogenic scrapie

In the 1930s several hundred cases of iatrogenic sheep scrapie were caused by the use of a batch of louping-ill vaccine prepared from scrapie contaminated, formalised sheep brain. Formalin does not completely inactivate scrapie agent.

Animal TSEs associated with feed

BSE and other SEs in domestic and captive wild BOVIDAE appear to be due to feeding concentrate feeds containing ruminant-derived meat and bone meal (see paras 2.2 and 2.3). TME has an origin in unprocessed ruminant tissues from sheep (or possibly cattle). The origin of FSE in domestic cats is presumptively from feed containing BSE agent, but the precise source is not known. The origin of FSE in captive wild FELIDAE is probably uncooked bovine carcase material containing central nervous tissue.

TSEs are infectious and transmissible, but do not appear to be naturally contagious except for scrapie and possibly CWD and SE in some captive wild ruminants. Some of the human diseases (GSS and familial CJD) may be inherited via mutations in an autosomal gene (the *PrP* gene) and polymorphisms in the same gene can modify the phenotype. In scrapie of sheep there is experimental evidence for maternal transmission via transferred embryos and by dosing with placenta. There is also epidemiological evidence supporting horizontal transmission of scrapie in sheep (presumed to result from consumption of placenta infected with the agent), and this may be a reason why scrapie is an endemic disease. The means of transmission of CWD and greater kudu SE is not known.

5.10 *Experimental host range for TSE agents*

Nervous tissue from cases of disease in natural hosts has been injected into a wide range of animal species. Transmission is regarded as positive when clinical disease and spongiform encephalopathy result in the recipient. Re-isolation of infectious agent from the brain by inoculation of the original host species or recipient species is a further criterion of success. The experimental host range of BSE agent determined in this way is shown at Table 5.1. Species barriers can be overcome when the factors described in para 5.6 are selected to maximise the effective exposure. Sometimes, however, even when this is done, transmissions are unsuccessful. Whether or not the barrier to transmission is absolute for a species is not known. The biological reasons for any difficulty in achieving transmissions might, in certain instances, be used to advantage; for example, in creating sheep genetically resistant to developing scrapie.

Table 5.1 Effect of inoculating BSE agent as bovine brain extract into eight species (minimum incubation period in months)

Species	Route of challenge	
	Oral	Parenteral
Mouse	Positive (15)	Positive (9.7)
Cattle	IP	Positive (18)
Sheep	Positive (18)	Positive (14)
Goat	Positive (31)	Positive (17)
Pig	IP	Positive (16)
Marmoset	ND	Positive (46)
Mink	Positive (15)	Positive (12)
Hamster	ND	Negative

ND = not done

IP = in progress

Adapted from: Bradley R. (1994) Bull. Soc. Vét. Prat. de France *78*, 339-366. Data provided by kind permission of Dr H Fraser, Mr J Foster, Mr G A H Wells, Mr M Dawson, Dr R Ridley and Dr M Robinson.

5.11 *Tissue assays in sheep with scrapie*

Natural scrapie of Suffolk sheep has been intensively studied by titrating tissues throughout the incubation period by mouse bioassay. No infectivity was detected until 10 months of age and then only in the gut and lymphoid tissue. It was not found in the CNS until about 2 years of age, at which time the animals were clinically healthy but infectivity titres had risen and plateaued in the lymphoreticular system (LRS). When the animals became clinically affected with scrapie at about 3½ years of age, the titre was highest in the brain, remained constant at a lower level in the LRS, and was not detected in most other tissues. At no time was it detected in milk, udder or muscle.

5.12 *Tissue assays in clinical cases of BSE and brain titrations in BSE and scrapie*

By contrast tests of cattle with symptomatic terminal BSE have (to date) detected infectivity only in central nervous tissue (brain and cervical spinal cord). Titrations in mice revealed mean titres of $10^{5.3}$ intracerebral ID_{50} mouse infectious units per gram of brainstem. The comparable mean titres in the medulla oblongata of terminally-affected Suffolk sheep with scrapie were $10^{5.6}$ per gram (Table 5.2).

No infectivity has been found in muscle, milk, udder, placenta, liver, kidney, blood, bone marrow, spleen, lymph nodes, semen and a range of other tissues from cows confirmed to have BSE (Table 5.3). Cattle have also been oro-nasally challenged with placenta derived from cattle clinically affected with BSE. Animals killed 2 years after exposure revealed no clinical or pathological evidence of BSE and all the remaining cattle remain healthy over 4 years after challenge.

5.13 *Pathogenesis, attack rate and concurrent assays/titrations in mice and cattle*

A study of the pathogenesis of BSE in cattle following oral challenge is in progress so that tissues for bioassay and/or titration can be sampled during the course of incubation. This study aims to identify those tissues which may become infected with the BSE agent, the temporal progression of infectivity and the infectivity titres reached during the incubation period. It cannot be conducted with naturally exposed animals because these cannot be identified and unlike in scrapie, there is no clear familial transmission of disease. Thirty cattle were dosed orally with 100g of brain at 4 months of age and there are 10 undosed controls. Starting at 6 months of age and at 4 month intervals thereafter, three challenged animals and one control are killed and 46 tissues collected for bioassay in mice. Preliminary results have shown that in the second and third kills (10 and 14 months of age, 6 and 10 months after challenge) the distal ileum contains infectivity. No clinical disease has yet occurred in any challenged calf, the oldest of which has reached 32 months of age.

Table 5.2 Infectivity titres (bioassayed in mice) in tissues from up to 9 Suffolk sheep (34-57 months old) and up to 3 goats (38-49 months old), at the clinical stage of natural scrapie, compared to the titres in tissues from 1 or more confirmed cases of BSE

Tissues	Titre (mean ±SEM of (n) samples) [a]				Titre [a]
	Scrapie sheep		Scrapie goats		BSE cattle
Category I					
Brain	5.6 ± 0.2	(51)	6.5 ± 0.2	(18)	5.3
Spinal cord	5.4 ± 0.3	(9)	6.1 ± 0.2	(6)	+ve
Category II					
Ileum	4.7 ± 0.1	(9)	4.6 ± 0.3	(3)	<2.0
Lymph nodes	4.2 ± 0.1	(45)	4.8 ± 0.1	(3)	<2.0
Proximal colon	4.5 ± 0.2	(9)	4.7 ± 0.2	(3)	<2.0
Spleen	4.5 ± 0.3	(9)	4.5 ± 0.1	(3)	<2.0
Tonsil	4.2 ± 0.4	(9)	5.1 ± 0.1	(3)	<2.0
Category III					
Sciatic nerve	3.1 ± 0.3	(9)	3.6 ± 0.3	(3)	<2.0
Distal colon	$< 2.7 \pm 0.2$	(9)	3.3 ± 0.5	(3)	<2.0
Thymus	2.2 ± 0.2	(9)	$< 2.3 \pm 0.2$	(3)	?.?
Bone marrow	$< 2.0 \pm 0.1$	(9)	< 2.0	(3)	<2.0
Liver	$< 2.0 \pm 0.1$	(9)	---		<2.0
Lung	< 2.0	(9)	$< 2.1 \pm 0.1$	(2)	<2.0
Pancreas	$< 2.1 \pm 0.1$	(9)	---		<2.0
Category IV					
Blood clot	< 1.0	(9)	<1.0	(3)	<1.0
Heart muscle	< 2.0	(9)	---		<2.0
Kidney	< 2.0	(9)	<2.0	(3)	<2.0
Mammary gland	<2.0	(7)	<2.0	(3)	<2.0
Milk	---		<1.0	(3)	?.?
Serum	---		<1.0	(3)	<1.0
Skeletal muscle	<2.0	(9)	<2.0	(1)	<2.0
Testis	<2.0	(1)	---		<2.0

The data are taken from the following sources: sheep scrapie, Hadlow *et al* (1982); goat scrapie, Hadlow *et al* (1980); BSE, Fraser *et al* (1992); Fraser & Foster (1994), these proceedings as Kimberlin (below). The classification of tissues is according to the CPMP Guidelines (EC, 1991).

[a]Titres are expressed as arithmetic means of log 10 mouse i/c. LD_{50}/g or ml of tissue (+ve > 2.0).
NOTE: None of the bovine tissues in categories II and III and no tissues in Category IV had any detectable infectivity. The values shown are maxima based on the limits of detectability of the bioassay in mice (calculated for 30μl of inoculum injected intracerebrally.

+ve = transmission positive but not titrated
?.?,--- = not done or not available

From: Kimberlin, R.H. (1994) A scientific evaluation of research into bovine spongiform encephalopathy (BSE). In: Transmissible Spongiform Encephalopathies. Proceedings of a Consultation on BSE with the Scientific Veterinary Committee of the Commission of the European Communities, held in Brussels, 14-15 September 1993. Editors R Bradley and B Marchant. CEC, Brussels, pp 455-477.

A parallel study (also using oral challenge) is underway to determine the attack rate (*ie* the percentage of animals succumbing to disease) at different doses (1g, 10g, 100g of brain once, or 100g on three occasions). This also is incomplete. A third study is in progress using, in separate experiments, cattle brain, spleen and pooled lymph nodes, each from pooled tissues of five cattle, which are being titrated (brain) or assayed at single low dilution (spleen and lymph nodes) in cattle and mice. In this way the sensitivity of the bioassay in mice will be compared with that in cattle by titrating in both species. Again no results are yet available.

Table 5.3 Lack of detectable infectivity in tissues (listed by anatomical group) of cattle with proven BSE

MOUSE CHALLENGE BY PARENTERAL (I/C I/P) INOCULATION

SPLEEN	SKELETAL MUSCLE M.DIAPHRAGMA M.MASSETER M.LONGISSIMUS M.SEMITENDINOSUS	LIVER KIDNEY PANCREAS	TESTIS PROSTATE SEMEN
LYMPH NODES MESENTERIC PREFEMORAL RETROPHARYNGEAL	BONE MARROW	OESOPHAGUS RETICULUM	OVARY UTERINE CARUNCLE PLACENTAL COTYLEDON
TONSIL	BUFFY COAT	RUMEN OESOPHAGEAL GROOVE PILLAR	AMNIOTIC FLUID ALLANTOIC FLUID
CAUDA EQUINA	SERUM		
PERIPHERAL NERVE N.SCIATICUS N.TIBIALIS ·N.SPLANCHNICUS	BLOOD CLOT	OMASUM ABOMASUM	
CEREBROSPINAL FLUID	FETAL CALF BLOOD	SMALL INTESTINE PROXIMAL DISTAL	
	MIDRUM FAT	COLON PROXIMAL DISTAL	
	UDDER	SKIN	
	HEART	LUNG	

Data courtesy of Dr H Fraser IAH, NPU Edinburgh

In addition, no detectable infectivity was found in milk and udder; spleen; placenta; carcase and mesenteric lymph nodes; or supramammary lymph nodes when fed in large quantities to susceptible mice (Middleton D J and Barlow R M (1993) Vet. Rec. *132*, 545-547).

5.14 *Other studies*

Four other major transmission studies are in progress. In one study, milk from cattle at early, middle and late lactation is fed to, or inoculated into susceptible mice. This milk study is an extension, on a broader scale, of one already completed in which no detectable infectivity for mice was present in either the milk or the mammary gland from which it was secreted. Another study is investigating natural maternal transmission in cattle (see para 5.16), and a third is examining the possibility of transmission of infection by embryo transfer (see para 5.18). Finally there is an experimental study of the effectiveness of various rendering procedures on BSE and scrapie agents (see para 5.19).

5.15 *Transmission from human tissues*

There have been few studies of experimental transmission from tissues of humans with CJD. However infectivity has been found in cases of kuru in brain, spinal cord, kidney, spleen and lymph node; and in human CJD in brain, cerebrospinal fluid, kidney, liver, lung and lymph nodes. There is also evidence for infection in pituitary gland, dura mater and cornea from iatrogenic disease incidents, but it might derive from brain tissue in the first two instances. The possibility of transmission from blood has been suggested but a case control study in the UK failed to show that blood transfusion is a risk factor for CJD. Transmissions are planned from sporadic cases of CJD to the same strains of mice used in BSE transmission studies. Transgenic mice expressing human PrP have been challenged with human brain from cases of CJD and studies are also in progress, or planned, using tissues and brain from BSE affected cattle and brain from scrapie affected sheep.

5.16 *Maternal transmission*

This is recognised as an established feature only in sheep scrapie. A major study of maternal transmission in BSE is underway, as recommended by Professor Southwood's Working Party. The objective of this study is to determine the occurrence and incidence of maternal transmission

in the BSE epidemic. 315 pairs of calves were purchased from farms in England and have been reared and kept in three assembled herds on MAFF experimental farms. Each pair consisted of a an exposed animal (that is, an offspring from a confirmed case) and a control calf. The control was a calf from the same herd and birth cohort whose dam was over 6 years of age and unaffected by BSE. All the selected cattle are being kept (without mating to avoid any possible spread of disease via placenta) until they are 7 years old. During this time regular clinical inspection for BSE is being undertaken (suspects are dealt with under the BSE Order). At the end of the study brains from all the cattle will be examined for evidence of spongiform encephalopathy. The study is being conducted blind and is into the fifth year of a 7 year study. To September 1994 29 cattle have been confirmed to have BSE but most, if not all, could have been exposed to a feed source of infection. Because of the continuous effect of feed as an alternative source of infection the study can only be evaluated by comparing the incidence of disease in the offspring of cases with that in controls and between members of a pair (to control for potential feed exposure) when the study is complete at the end of 1996.

5.17 *Embryo transfer (ET) in sheep*

Many infectious agents do not transmit disease via ET provided that the strict protocols of the International ET Society (IETS) (which includes washing embryos ten times) are followed. Therefore ET can be an important way to minimise the risks of infectious agents being spread to offspring or recipients and from country to country as when germplasm is imported. Reports of an ET experiment in the USA where sheep embryos were washed only three times have so far shown no transmission of scrapie to recipients or offspring. However, the experiment was confounded by a number of uncontrolled variables and had a positive control group with a low incidence of disease (*ie* a group consisting of scrapie inoculated donors and inoculated recipients). Another ET study in sheep has been reported in which there was transmission of scrapie in offspring derived from the embryos of scrapie-inoculated dams which were transferred into scrapie-free and scrapie-resistant recipients. In this study embryos were deliberately not washed according to IETS protocols, in order to maximise the chance of transmission - which did, in fact, occur in six out of six genetically susceptible (*Sip sAsA*) ewes (Foster *et al* (1992) Vet. Rec. *130*, 341-343). The experiment is being repeated with embryos washed in accordance with normal practice to determine whether or not this removes scrapie contamination.

5.18 *Embryo transfer in cattle*

The objectives of the ET experiment are to determine whether embryos derived from BSE-infected cattle are infective for recipient dams or progeny. The design of this experiment is shown in Figure 5.1.

The donors were clinical cases from the field and recipients were imported cattle from New Zealand, a country with neither BSE nor scrapie. These cattle are maintained in quarantine on a MAFF experimental farm. All embryos were treated according to the IETS protocol before transfer or inoculation. Embryos unsuitable for transfer were pooled and inoculated into mice, as were uterine flushings. The current status of the study is shown in Table 5.4.

BSE has not occurred so far in any cows given embryos, or offspring derived from those embryos, neither has spongiform encephalopathy occurred in any mice given embryos or uterine flushings - the study will not be complete until 2001. Though the thrust of this experiment is to provide data to facilitate trade in embryos it is also strategically very important. This is because if BSE unexpectedly becomes an endemic disease in some herds, a proven embryo transfer technique could be used to retrieve valuable cattle genes whilst removing the risk of infection. In this event the data would be extremely useful.

Figure 5.1 ET - Fate of embryos and uterine flushings

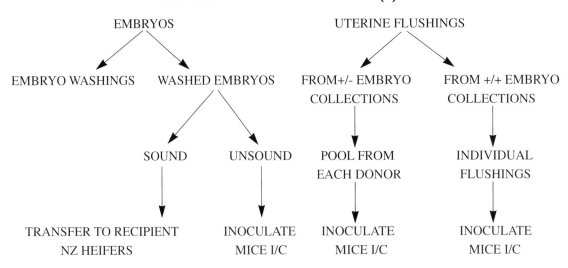

The donor cows (+) were field cases of BSE brought to CVL Weybridge. Cows were inseminated either with semen from bulls with confirmed BSE (+) or, semen collected from bulls born before 1980 (-). After artificial insemination embryos were collected by flushing the uterus a few days later, according to IETS protocols and freezing them in liquid nitrogen. Brains from these cows were examined to confirm BSE. The recipient cows (-) were imported into the UK from New Zealand to a quarantine farm where sound embryos, collected at CVL, were transferred. The recipient cows and the offspring resulting from embryo transfer will be clinically examined frequently and kept for 7 years before killing and examination of the brain for BSE. Flushings and unsound embryos are inoculated into mice, clinically examined through their lifespan and brains will be examined at death.

Table 5.4 Current status of cattle embryo transfer experiment

CATTLE	
- BSE CONFIRMED DONOR COWS	167
- TRANSFERABLE QUALITY EMBRYOS	1095
- RECIPIENTS EXPOSED TO EMBRYOS	347
- CALVES BORN:	
SPRING 1992 AND REARED TO JUNE 1994	99
SPRING 1993 AND REARED TO JUNE 1994	107
AUTUMN 1993 AND REARED TO JUNE 1994	44
MICE	
- NON-TRANSFERABLE QUALITY EMBRYOS/OVA	1293
CATTLE EMBRYOS/OVA INOCULATED INTO MICE	860
- FLUSHINGS FROM BSE-CONFIRMED DONOR COWS	481
UTERINE FLUSHINGS (SOME MULTIPLE) INOCULATED INTO MICE	40

As at JUNE 1994

Data courtesy of Dr A E Wrathall.

5.19 *Rendering study*

The probable origins of the BSE epidemic lie in changes to the methods of rendering ruminant waste from abattoirs, butchers' and knackers' in the early 1980s (Figure 5.2). The changes are thought to have increased the exposure of cattle to scrapie (and BSE) agents via dietary meat and bone meal to the point where clinical disease ensued. In Great Britain the initial source of infection was probably scrapie-infected material from sheep and, from 1984 onwards, from cattle infected with BSE agent. This lasted at least until July 1988 when the ruminant feed ban was introduced. Such an exposure to scrapie has probably not occurred in other countries due to the different ratio of sheep to cattle and the lower incidence of the disease. Nevertheless, the European Commission, which had a responsibility for developing rules for the safe trading of commodities including meat and bone meal, set up an experiment in collaboration with MAFF, IAH (NPU), the European Renderers Association (EURA) and Prosper de Mulder (UK). The experiment used a small scale, pilot rendering plant to determine the effectiveness of representative rendering systems used throughout the EC to

Figure 5.2 Outline of commercial rendering

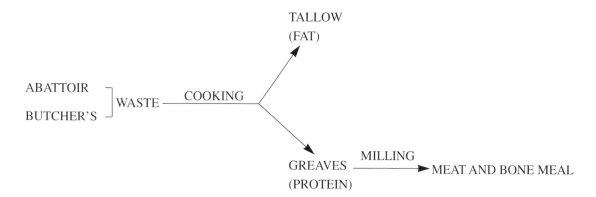

decontaminate abattoir waste. Bones and intestines were spiked with:

▲ BSE from UK cattle brains or

▲ scrapie from UK sheep brains.

▲ A third study was proposed with sheep scrapie from mainland Europe sheep brains but no brains have yet been collected.

The design is complex and a simplified version is shown at Figure 5.3 and with results at Table 5.5.

Progress to date has determined the amount of infectivity (by mouse bioassay) in the BSE spike and shown that some methods employing minimal heat and time which are used in Great Britain and in some other Member States are ineffective in inactivating the infectivity in the spiked material (Table 5.5). These methods have been banned by the European Commission for processing ruminant material (with certain exceptions). No infectivity was found in the tallow prepared from the spiked material. Many of the mice injected with MBM and tallow prepared using other methods are still alive. The UK scrapie-spiked material has been rendered (cooked). The scrapie spike and MBM samples have been inoculated into mice. As the brains from mainland European sheep with scrapie have not been provided alternative approaches are under discussion for the third phase of these studies.

5.20 *Agent inactivation*

Other important studies on agent inactivation are being undertaken at the NPU using conventional autoclaving, a variety of inactivating chemicals and a laboratory scale hydrocarbon solvent rendering system.

The results of these studies showed that BSE and scrapie agents respond similarly to chemical and

Figure 5.3 Experimental study of inactivation of BSE agent by various pilot scale rendering procedures

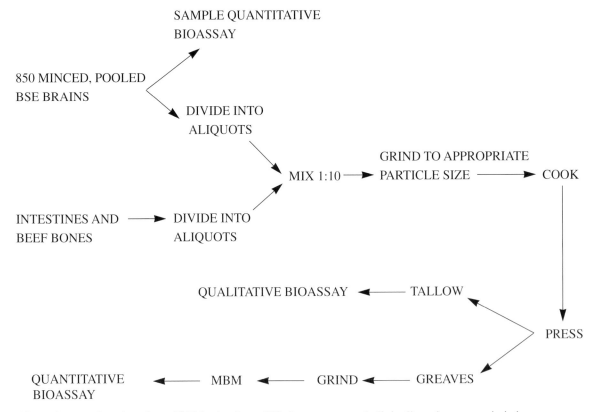

Note: A second study using c3000 brains from UK sheep suspected clinically to have scrapie is in progress using a similar protocol. In each study the objective is to determine the reduction in titre in the final products (meat and bone meal and tallow) compared with that in the start material (pooled brains).

After Woodgate S L (1994) Rendering systems and BSE agent deactivation. Livestock Prod. Sci. Special Issue *38*, 47-50.

physical inactivation procedures. They are both resistant to inactivation by formaldehyde but sodium hypochlorite is an effective decontaminant. Dichloroisocyanurate, which can yield similar chlorine concentrations to hypochlorite, does not completely inactivate BSE agent. Sodium hydroxide at 1M or 2M concentration is a useful decontaminating reagent but does not completely inactivate large amounts of infectivity.

The lower end of the range (134°C) recommended for decontaminating scrapie agent by porous load autoclaving may permit residual infectivity to remain in both scrapie or BSE challenge studies.

The single message that comes from these studies is that BSE agent behaves like scrapie agent in being highly resistant to decontamination, though effective and practical methods of disinfection are available. Nevertheless the best advice on the problem of contamination is to avoid or minimise contamination in the first place, or destroy contaminated material (such as surgical instruments or tissues) rather than rely on decontamination procedures being 100% effective.

5.21 *Risk assessment, CJD surveillance and monitoring*

The SEAC has continuously reviewed the new data emerging from the epidemiological and other studies on the BSE epidemic with a view to making a judgement of the risks to man and other species. The risk to man from BSE depends on the inherent risk that the BSE agent is a human pathogen, which cannot yet be evaluated, and on the level of exposure to the pathogen, which can. Since scrapie

Table 5.5 Summary of various processing conditions in pilot scale rendering experiment

Type	Particle diameter (mm)	Fat content	Process time (min)	Achieved end temperature (^{0}C)	Bioassays Meal (M) Tallow (T)	Pass/ Fail
Batch atmospheric	150	Natural (N)	150	121	(M)	Pass
Continuous atmospheric	30	N	*50* 125	*112/122* 123/139	*M* M	*Fail* Pass
Continuous atmospheric	30	High (H) 1:1	30/120	136/137	M	Pass
Continuous vacuum	*10*	*H 4:1*	*10* *40*	*120* *121*	*M T** *M*	*Fail* *Fail*
Continuous wet rendering	20 (1:5:4)	N	120/240	101/119	M	Pass
Batch pressure cook raw	30/50	N	28/30	133/136/145	M T	Pass

Raw materials 861 BSE suspect cow forebrains (10%) mixed with intestines and beef bones (90%) - ratios 1:3:6 or 1:5:4
Mouse bioassays - 1) mixed raw material, 2) meat and bone meal (M), 3) tallow (T)

Note: 'Type' (column 1) refers to major rendering processes used in the EU and elsewhere. The next four columns refer to the parameters used in the study and representative of those used by renderers in the EU. Column 6 indicates which samples were bioassayed in mice. The processes in italics are those in which infectivity was found in meat and bone meal after rendering and which were banned by the CEC. *Note that no infectivity was found in tallow after continuous vacuum processing.

Adapted from: Woodgate S L (1994) Rendering systems and BSE agent deactivation. Livestock Production Science. Special Issue. *38*, 47-50.

Taylor D M (1994) Personal communication.

was first clearly described in the literature of the 18th century there has been no epidemiological linkage of the disease, or indeed any animal TSE, with human disease, or vice versa. This does not prove there is no risk, but it suggests that any risk is probably small. To check that it is, the only means is to continue the in-progress CJD surveillance programme. This is because any unaccountable rise in incidence of CJD might hypothetically derive from animals. The logical target origin would be BSE, because it is a new disease and has occurred at a high incidence.

Twelve years after the first effective exposure of cows to BSE agent no such cases in man have been identified. Two recent cases of sporadic CJD in British dairy farmers are regarded as chance occurrences, not least because the clinical signs and other features are entirely consistent with a diagnosis of sporadic CJD. They are not like those in kuru or in peripherally exposed iatrogenic cases, which experts consider would be the more likely clinical presentation of BSE-derived infection. Our conclusion therefore is that, as the Southwood Working Party determined, taking all the available evidence together, the risk to man from BSE is remote. Nevertheless, advice given by them and this Committee has been aimed at reducing exposure of humans to the BSE agent. Long term this is achieved by the ruminant protein feed ban which is already showing evidence of success in eliminating BSE in the cattle population and preventing new infections of all ruminants via feed. In the short term the compulsory notification, slaughter and complete destruction of clinically suspect BSE cases, together with the SBO ban (including the extension to include the distal ileum and thymus of calves under 6 months of age used for human consumption) is protecting consumers from any significant exposure.

We are also content that the bioassay of tissues from confirmed, affected BSE cattle realistically reflects the tissues in which the agent may be present in significant quantity (brain and spinal cord) and those in which it is not detected (muscle, milk, liver, kidney, heart, testis, ovary, semen, tonsil, spleen, gut lymphoid tissues and many others). We believe that these measures and others relating to biologicals prepared from bovine tissues, or used in their manufacture (another potential source of BSE infection for man and animals), are sufficient with current knowledge to satisfactorily protect human and animal health.

Although we do not know for certain the source of FSE in domestic cats, all the evidence (temporal and geographic occurrence of the disease, and agent strain typing) points to a feed source and probable origin from BSE rather than from scrapie. The initial cases of SE in all the captive wild ruminant species, except the scimitar-horned oryx, were exposed to the same infected feed as cattle. The origin of infection in the scimitar-horned oryx and subsequent cases in greater kudu and eland is not known. The wild FELIDAE affected by FSE have been exposed to raw, central nervous tissue from potentially BSE-affected/infected cattle carcases. 'Species jumping' is not an appropriate term to use since all these species have been exposed, probably via feed, provided 'artificially' by man. Indeed without man's interference BSE itself would never have occurred. In conclusion, therefore, our scientific assessment is that the risk to man and other species from BSE is remote because the control measures now in place are adequate to eliminate or reduce any risk to a negligible level. We do however point out that any species exposed already and before any bans were effective could be incubating disease, and therefore continuous monitoring is very important until any possible incubation period has been exceeded.

Reading list

BAKER H F, RIDLEY R M AND WELLS G A H. (1993) Experimental transmission of BSE and scrapie to the common marmoset. Vet. Rec. *132*, 403-406.

BRADLEY R. (1994) Embryo transfer and its potential role in control of scrapie and bovine spongiform encephalopathy. Livestock Production Science. Special Issue *38*, 51-59.

BROWN P, GIBBS C J, RODGERS-JOHNSON P, ASHER D M, SULIMA M P, BACOTE A, GOLDFARB L G AND GAJDUSEK D C. (1994) Human spongiform encephalopathy: The National Institutes of Health series of 300 cases of experimentally transmitted disease. Ann. Neurol. *35*, 513-529.

DAWSON M, WELLS G A H AND PARKER B N J. (1990) Prelminary evidence of the experimental transmissibility of bovine spongiform encephalopathy to cattle. Vet. Rec. *126,* 112-113.

DAWSON M, WELLS G A H, PARKER B N J AND SCOTT A C. (1990) Primary parenteral transmission of bovine spongiform encephalopathy to the pig. Vet. Rec. *127,* 138.

FOOTE W C, CLARK W, MACIULIS A, CALL J W, HOURRIGAN J, EVANS R C, MARSHALL M R AND de CAMP M. (1993) Prevention of scrapie transmission in sheep, using embryo transfer. Am. J. Vet. Res. *54,* 1863-1868.

FOSTER J D, McKELVEY W A C, MYLNE M J A, WILLIAMS A, HUNTER N, HOPE J AND FRASER H. (1992) Studies on maternal transmission of scrapie in sheep by embryo transfer. Vet. Rec. *130,* 341-343.

FRASER H, BRUCE M E, CHREE A, McCONNELL I AND WELLS G A H. (1992) Transmission of bovine spongiform encephalopathy and scrapie to mice. J. Gen. Virol. *73,* 1891-1897.

MIDDLETON D J AND BARLOW R M. (1993) Failure to transmit bovine spongiform encephalopathy to mice by feeding them with extraneural tissues of affected cattle. Vet. Rec. *132,* 545-547.

TAYLOR D M. (1991) Inactivation of the unconventional agents of scrapie, bovine spongiform encephalopathy and Creutzfeldt-Jakob disease. J. Hosp. Inf. *18,* (A) 141-146.

WELLS G A H, DAWSON M, HAWKINS S A C, GREEN R B, DEXTER I, FRANCIS M E, SIMMON M M, AUSTIN A R AND HORIGAN M W. (1994) Infectivity in the ileum of cattle challenged orally with bovine spongiform encephalopathy. Vet. Rec. *135,* 40-41.

WOODGATE S L. (1994) Rendering systems and BSE agent deactivation. Livestock Production Science. Special Issue. *38,* 47-50.

WRATHALL A E AND BROWN K F D. (1991) Embryo transfer, semen, scrapie and BSE. In: Sub-acute Spongiform Encephalopathies. Editors R Bradley, M Savey and B Marchant. Kluwer Academic Publishers, Dordrecht, pp 243-253.

Molecular Studies

6.1 *Introduction*

Scrapie was thought at one time to be due to a virus infection, but subsequent detailed study showed that the scrapie agent did not have the characteristic properties of a virus. For example, no specific antibodies or immunity were found. Also it was remarkably heat resistant and its apparent diameter determined by ionizing irradiation was remarkably small. In fact an important unanswered question for modern biology is the nature of the causative agents of the TSEs. Certain basic findings need to be explained - replication, for example, and the fact that different strains of scrapie exhibit marked differences in the incubation period and in the distribution of lesions in mice of the same genotype. The same strain of agent shows different incubation periods and lesion profiles in mice of different genotypes. These agent strains usually breed true, but mutant strains can be selected on passage across the 'species barrier', when infectious material from one species is injected into another. These properties (replication, strain variation and mutation) are usually based on nucleic-acid containing genomes. However, attempts to show the presence and role of such nucleic acids, either DNA or RNA, have not succeeded. Indeed most new positive results concern the PrP^{Sc} and this will be discussed first.

6.2 *Partially protease resistant protein (PrP)*

In a search for a scrapie virus it was found that detergent extracts of scrapie-affected brain contained characteristic fibrils called scrapie associated fibrils or SAF (Figure 1.6). These fibrils are derived from a host protein (PrP) with a molecular ratio (M_r) of 33-35kDa (see para 1.13, Figure 1.3), modified to partially resist protease digestion. This partially protease resistant protein can also be detected and characterised chemically, for example in stained electrophoresis gels. The M_r of the derived protein is about 27-30kDa and is also known as PrP 27-30. It can be identified by immunoblotting using antiserum made by injecting SAF protein into a heterologous species such as a rabbit.

This PrP has been studied in great detail, particularly by Dr S B Prusiner and his associates in various laboratories round the world. It is now known that it is the product of a gene that codes for a normal cellular protein - called PrP^C, and that this is converted into PrP^{Sc}, the partially protease resistant form found associated with disease, by some form of post-translational processing which remains undefined but may involve the formation of non-covalent bonds. The protein has been sequenced, and it is known to be glycosylated, and to be myristylated at one end (see Figure. 3.1). It thus has affinities with membrane proteins but its function in normal cells is unknown. The protein is anchored to the neuronal surface by glycosylphosphatidylinositol (the GPI anchor) suggesting a role in cell signalling or adhesion. Some recent research by the Prion Disease Group at St Mary's Hospital Medical School, London has revealed that brain slices from PrP null mice have weakened gamma-aminobutyric acid type A (GABA$_A$) receptor-mediated fast inhibition and impaired long-term potentiation. In other words there is an impairment to the normal inhibition of transmission between neurons. The authors suggest the epileptiform activity seen in CJD and scrapie-affected mice may be due to this weakened inhibition at synapses (junctions between some cells) and argue that loss of function of PrP^C may contribute to the neuronal degeneration seen in CJD-like diseases.

PrP is present early in embryonic life but does not appear to be essential for normal development and function in mice as transgenic mice (see below) in which the *PrP* gene has been deleted apparently develop normally. Its sequence is well conserved in mammalian species and there is some (30%) sequence homology with an avian protein that co-purifies with acetylcholine receptor-inducing activity: all the structural features of mammalian PrP were found in the chicken protein derived from brain.

Figure 6.1 More detailed representation of the biosynthesis of PrP^C and PrP^{Sc} (compare with Figure 4.1)

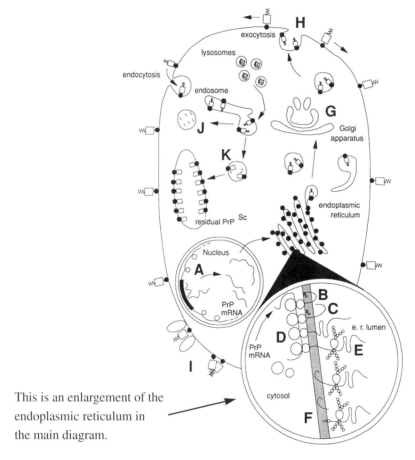

This is an enlargement of the endoplasmic reticulum in the main diagram.

mRNA is transcribed in the nucleus (**A**) and passed out to the cytoplasm, where it is translated by ribosomes at the endoplasmic reticulum (**B**). At this stage the N-terminal signal peptide is removed (**C**) to form the mature N-terminus (**D**), the sugars are added at N-linked glycosylation sites (**E**) and the C-terminal peptide is removed at the time that the GPI tail is added (**F**). The protein moves through the Golgi on its way to the surface (**G**) at which time the high mannose oligomers become trimmed and replaced with the mature sugar residues. PrP is released to the surface (**H**), and, through interaction with itself and/or other proteins, may form higher order structures (**I**). In uninfected cells PrP^C is turned over by internalisation and lysosomal degradation (**J**). Whether endosomal recycling to the Golgi takes place is not known. For as yet unknown reasons, in infected cells PrP^{Sc} is not degraded and accumulates in the cell (**K**). A proportion of PrP^{Sc} is found to be partially digested, suggesting that it is exposed to proteolytic enzymes in passing through the lysosomes.

From: Bennett A D, Birkett C R and Bostock C J. (1992) Molecular biology of scrapie-like agents. Rev. sci. tech. Off. int. Epiz. *11*, 569-603.

Research has revealed the cellular sites of formation of PrP^{Sc} and its processing (trafficking) through the cell organelles to the plasma membrane (Figures 4.1 and 6.1).

It is clear that PrP is closely involved in the disease process. For example, it accumulates extracellularly in those areas of the CNS in which morphological changes develop, and often ahead of these changes. The mechanisms that cause vacuolation have not been defined though it has been found that ubiquitin and Tau proteins accumulate along with PrP and lysosomal markers in association with primary vesicles.

6.3 *Tissue culture*

It is difficult to do certain types of experiment by study of whole brain and progress would be greatly accelerated if *in vitro* systems were available in which cultures of uniformly affected cells could be studied biochemically and morphologically. Tissue cultures have been prepared using a neural cell line which differentiates in the presence of nerve growth factor (NGF) and then replicates scrapie strains, but they need to be made more productive, if possible, to be fully exploited in this way. Already scrapie agent strains have been found which grow well in cultured cells, cause no apparent damage but alter the formation of neurotransmitters. Tissue culture methods, for example using scrapie-infected neuroblastoma cells, have revealed much about the intracellular trafficking of PrP *in vitro*.

Tissue culture methods may enable us to determine if various chemical/drug treatments influence the formation, proteolysis and accumulation of PrP^{Sc} in a favourable way. In the long term particular drugs might be used to treat human patients, and particularly those who are at risk from developing CJD as a result of iatrogenic exposure or being related to familial CJD cases and are carrying the relevant *PrP* gene mutation. The dye, Congo red, has already been identified as one chemical which interferes with PrP^{Sc} accumulation. A variety of other neural and non-neural cell lines are being investigated as possible *in vitro* systems. It might even be possible to develop sensitive and convenient assays for detecting TSE infectivity using, for example, cell lines developed from

transgenic animals or from sheep which are genetically susceptible to certain scrapie strains that occur in the field.

A recent paper (Kocisko *et al* 1994) has reported the conversion of PrP^C to PrP^{Sc} in a cell-free system of substantially purified constituents. This type of study may enable us to understand more clearly how the conversion operates. If this experiment can be repeated it will provide persuasive evidence that PrP^{Sc} can be formed *in vitro* by protein-protein interaction. The method might then be used to show whether the 'species barrier' and the effect of pathogenic mutations depend on the efficiency with which one PrP interacts with another. However, to show that PrP^{Sc} can act as an infectious agent it will be necessary to show, in a rigorously purified system, that it can convert PrP^C efficiently when present as a minor component of a mixture, rather than as an excess as in the present system. Furthermore, mouse cells producing PrP^{Sc} in tissue culture failed to do so when they were transfected and produced a heterologous PrP with a sequence differing by one amino acid from that of mouse PrP.

6.4 *Transgenics*

A relatively new method, namely the creation of transgenic animals, has also been exploited. By inserting foreign genes into mouse embryos and growing these into adults it is feasible to develop new strains of animals that possess the foreign gene in the germline and express the gene product in tissues. Again, in order to test whether it is the sequence of the *PrP* gene that produces the donor species effect when scrapie is transferred from one species to another, transgenic animals have been injected with scrapie material from different species. The results of studies using mice and hamsters show that recipient animals expressing PrP like that of the donor animal tend to have incubation periods like those in the donor and unlike those in the non-transgenic recipient (Table 6.1).

6.5 *Gene sequencing*

The *PrP* of patients with familial, iatrogenic or sporadic CJD, GSS, and fatal familial insomnia has been sequenced. Interesting differences from the *PrP* gene of normal subjects have been found except in the sporadic patients; either single amino acid substitutions, apparently as the result of point mutations, or changes in the number of so called octa-peptide repeats (illustrated in Figure 1.7). As the figure shows, these sequences are associated with disease and various patterns are emerging. For example, a proline to leucine change at codon 102 is associated with cases of ataxic GSS. Other forms of GSS are associated with mutations at codons 117, 198 and 217 (Figure 3.1). This is forceful support for other evidence that shows that the *PrP* gene structure is of prime importance in the TSEs. For example, the genes associated with susceptibility to scrapie in sheep and in mice (see above) are closely associated with, if not identical to, the *PrP* genes of those species, and *PrP* gene-ablated 'null' mice are another example.

6.6 *The nature of the agents of TSEs*

The problem of the nature of TSE 'agents' resembles that of the fierce debates of previous decades about the nature of viruses. For instance Northrop focused on viruses being proteins to be analysed and understood as proteins, and Delbruck focused on their ability to replicate and behave as genetic entities. A similar debate began decades ago with a wide range of hypotheses that have now been abandoned, including some proposals that the scrapie agent might be a carbohydrate. Of the three main original contenders of agent structure (see para 1.19) two currently dominate the scene. These are the prion and virino hypotheses. While the third (virus hypothesis) has not been disproved, there is less support for it now than formerly. A hypothetical concept has been evolved to attempt to meld the prion and virino hypotheses into one. This is a 'Unified Theory' and uses new terms such as 'apoprion' and 'coprion' which together form the 'holoprion'. The apoprion is PrP^{Sc}. The coprion is a nucleic acid of which many variants exist, and determines strain-specific characteristics. Normally they are closely associated but are also present in uninfected host cells. When the apoprion enters a cell devoid of coprion it may recruit a cellular RNA as the coprion. The presence of PrP^{Sc} is required to promote the replication of the coprion RNA. Thus the apoprion can be propagated and cause disease and the coprion can enhance the effectiveness of propagation. This hypothesis has not gained much support.

Each of these concepts accommodates some well-attested features of TSEs, but none is free of difficulties. However it is a tantalising problem, the solution of which offers the chance of explaining an

Table 6.1 Modification of the incubation period of scrapie in 3 groups of transgenic (Tg) mice carrying the hamster (Ha) *PrP* gene

Species and strain	Scrapie⁺ animals	Mean incubation (days ± SEM)
Hamsters (non-Tg)	48/48	77±1
Mice (Tg)		
Tg 81 (30 - 50 copies)	22/22	75 ± 2
Tg 71 (4 - 6 copies)	14/15	172 ± 4
Tg 54* (Ha minigene)	0/15	> 731

⁺ = Figures show ratio of affected to inoculated animals
* = Effectively a 'control', intronless transgene which cannot code for Ha PrP

Animals were inoculated parenterally with scrapie agent and observed for disease.

Modified from: Scott M, Foster D, Mirenda C, Serban D, Coufal F, Walchli M, Torchia M, Groth D, Carlson G, DeArmond S J, Westaway D and Prusiner S B. (1989) Transgenic mice expressing hamster prion protein produce species-specific scrapie infectivity and amyloid plaques. Cell *59*, 847-857.

aspect of biology of which we are ignorant at the moment. There is also the opportunity to develop useful knowledge, such as novel diagnostic tests and targets for drug action, as well as a better understanding of other neurodegenerative diseases, for instance Alzheimer's disease.

6.7 *Protein only hypothesis*

Many laboratories favour some variant of the 'prion hypothesis' which will be reviewed first. All agree that the *PrP* gene and its protein product PrP play a central role in these diseases but this does not necessarily indicate the chemical nature of the agent. However, the prion hypothesis is that the modified form of the *PrP* gene product is the sole constituent of the infectious agent. Early studies suggested a correspondence between the presence and concentration of PrP^{Sc} and infectivity. For instance, they appear together in tissues during the course of an infection. When PrP is purified from brain the peak of infectivity and of PrP are often found in the same fractions. This is quite striking when very structure-specific methods, such as immunoaffinity purification are used. However, in all these experiments the bioassay for infectivity is not as precise as protein measurements so only large differences can be confidently detected.

Also it is possible that the association between PrP and infectivity is fortuitous because the agent is very sticky. Indeed there are experiments in which infectivity and PrP^{Sc} concentrations seemed to diverge quite widely. For instance when mice treated with amphotericin showed delayed accumulation of PrP^{Sc} the increase of infectivity was unaffected. A similar situation was reported in a recent study of salivary glands from mice experimentally infected with murine CJD where infectivity decreased as PrP concentration increased. It has also been claimed that infectivity and PrP can be, at least partly, separated by purification. There are always problems in interpreting such experiments *eg* some difference might be due to a degree of aggregation of infectivity rather than concentration, and the results are not always reproducible. However, it does appear that though some PrP^{Sc} is necessary for infectivity, much of it is not.

Another approach is to look for specific evidence that PrP^{Sc} alone is infectious. It is very difficult to exclude all possibility of contamination of PrP^{Sc} preparations so the *PrP* gene has been cloned and expressed; but it is not practical to ensure that it is glycosylated and myristylated* in a completely normal way or that the modification (from PrP^{C} to PrP^{Sc} for instance) can be made to occur exactly as it does within the cell. So attempts to make an infectious PrP in this way would be important if they succeeded, but not surprising if they did not, and so far no successes have been reported.

As mentioned above, a *PrP* gene can be introduced into a mouse so that all the progeny mice carry it and express the gene product - so called transgenic mice. Thus mice that overexpress a *PrP* mutant (GSS codon 102) gene have been produced and have in due course developed spongiform changes showing yet again the importance of PrP. However, even though GSS seems to be inherited, it is also transmissible experimentally to primates. Therefore brain extracts from these mice were tested for the presence of infectious agent and some positive results were obtained when inoculated into other mice and hamsters. However, there is some doubt about this, so this experiment needs independent verification.

One of the problems with the prion theory is that it infers that proteins can somehow 'propagate' themselves, and current biology considers that only nucleic acids replicate in living cells. However, it has been suggested that PrP^{Sc} has the property of inducing a conformational change in PrP^{C} in the host animal. This change is associated with partial protease resistance, the accumulation of PrP^{Sc} and the acquisition of infectivity. There is no evidence of what that change amounts to chemically, and it is probably a non-covalent conformational change. Another problem with the basic hypothesis is that it cannot readily explain the key issues of agent strain variation and mutation. For example attempts have been made to examine the difference in the biological properties of the 263K and 139H strains

---

* Note: Several cell and viral membrane proteins have a myristic acid group covalently attached directly to their polypeptide backbone. In PrP the myristate group is attached indirectly via the hydroxyl group of glycerol in the GPI anchor at the C-terminus of the protein.

in golden hamsters in terms of differences in glycosylation of PrP^{Sc}. However, recent studies using very sensitive methods have failed to find differences in patterns of glycosylation or other types of post-translational modification. Consequently the prion hypothesis has been modified to suggest that strain variation and mutation involve conformational (non-covalent) changes, but these are less convincing in explaining these phenomena.

However, a non-covalent conformational change in PrP^{C} may be all that is needed to account for the formation of PrP^{Sc}, which is apparently synthesized with the same amount of mRNA as in normal cells. Unlike PrP^{C}, PrP^{Sc} would then not be catabolised and would therefore accumulate. There are examples of protein-protein interactions which lead to structural and functional changes in a normal gene product; one such example is p53. Some groups have seen a close analogy between TSE and amyloidosis, and indeed there is some evidence that intracerebral injection into marmosets of extract of Alzheimer's disease brain is followed after some years by the appearance of typical amyloid plaques, but not of neurofibrillary tangles or of clinical disease. Evidence is being sought that altered PrP can induce the build up of arrays of molecules, but so far attempts to induce such changes in test tube systems have not succeeded. One new theory - the frame shifting hypothesis - suggests that PrP^{C} and PrP^{Sc} are chemically different due to frame shifting which results in amino acid differences in PrP^{Sc} and opportunities for crystallisation. However, other studies show that the amino acid sequence is the same for both forms of the protein and therefore the differences are post-translational. However, frame shifting could produce a very small proportion of PrP^{Sc} which might be associated with infectivity.

6.8   Nucleic acid

The main argument against the virino and virus theories is that no specific nucleic acid has been found in highly purified, infectious preparations. Although highly purified PrP^{Sc} does in fact contain small amounts of nucleic acid, this is apparently not of uniform size as one would expect if it were derived from a typical virus or viroid. Nevertheless one worker has found distinct bands of nucleic acid in preparations that are claimed to be infectious, and these bands may be derived from the agent genome. These observations are being independently investigated.

A recent publication reports the presence of small virus-like structures in fractions from experimental hamster scrapie brain. They are extremely small for a conventional virus but do have morphological features of small pentagonal viruses. They have a uniform size of 10-12nm diameter. The smallest virus known has a diameter of 18nm. The structures are found in preparations prepared for the examination of fibrils (SAF) by electron microscopy. It is premature, as the authors state, to consider that these structures are the elusive scrapie agent, but the observation will promote research to see if they exist in naturally occurring spongiform encephalopathies and to further characterise them.

It has been confirmed that the infectivity in scrapie preparations is resistant to nuclease digestion, but it is important to realise that the infectivity of most viruses is resistant to nucleases, because the nucleic acid is tightly associated with protein and within the virus particle. Furthermore, it is necessary to be aware of the limited quantitation that is possible with TSEs. It may be that there are substantial falls in infectivity when treated with a reagent, eg lipid solvent, yet because some infectivity survives treatment the result of the test is reported as 'resistant to treatment' but one tenfold dilution fall in titre means that a full 90% of infectivity has actually been lost. Finally it has been calculated that there is probably enough nucleic acid in purified PrP to account for the infectivity shown.

In the absence of direct chemical evidence for a genomic nucleic acid, an indirect approach to the problem arises from the evidence for mutation of scrapie strains. One might treat strains with carefully graded doses of specific nucleic acid mutagens and so look for the appearance of new mutants. Such work is now in progress.

Recent evidence from analysis of purified hamster scrapie preparations by return refocusing gel electrophoresis revealed nucleic acids up to 1100 nucleotides long. The method specifically concentrates heterogeneous nucleic acids which would otherwise be dispersed within the gel. If a scrapie-specific nucleic acid were homogeneous in size such a molecule would be <80 nucleotides long at a particle to infectivity ratio near unity. If however it were heterogeneous it would have to include molecules smaller than 240 nucleotides. Treatment with Benzonase, an enzyme which degrades DNA and RNA, did not destroy infectivity, but the studies did not completely exclude the existence of a nucleic acid.

6.9 *Biochemical alterations in scrapie-like diseases*

A wide range of clinical biochemical studies of body fluids and tissues from humans or animals with TSEs has been undertaken. None has revealed a specific component that is uniquely associated with the disease. However, there are two promising lines of enquiry. The first involves the analysis of cerebrospinal fluid (CSF) from clinical human patients who were later confirmed to have CJD. Essentially the method involves two dimensional (2-D) electrophoresis. The profiles of normal patients and those of affected patients have been compared and show additional proteins to be present in the latter. These studies have revealed 931 different 'spots' which can be related to <200 different proteins or their post-translational variants. These methods are now being applied to CSF from healthy cattle and those with BSE. The methods and instrumentation are continually improving so that the precision of the database from normal individuals can be enhanced and so comparisons can be made in different laboratories.

The second analysis, initially developed in France, involves the electrochemical analysis of urine from human patients with CJD, sheep with scrapie and cattle with BSE. In the animal diseases analyses have given encouraging results with sheep with scrapie (in France) and with laboratory-housed natural cases of BSE in the UK. Studies on herd mates of BSE cases in the field have not been so successful. The method is cumbersome and capricious and only useful for small numbers of samples in the laboratory. The method employs cyclical voltametry. An induced signal from repeated sweeps of increasing and decreasing potential is applied to reducible and oxidisable

components in the sample which then give rise to 'peaks' on the voltamogram at potentials specific for the low molecular weight molecule that is oxidised or reduced. Attempts are now being made to isolate the major redox component from large volumes of urine so that the metabolites with a profile specific for disease can be identified. This may permit the development of a more appropriate analytical method which might be useful for field use once the sensitivity and specificity are characterised.

Reading list

BANISSI-SABOURDY C, PLANQUES B, DAVID J P, JEANNIN C, POTEL M, BIZIEN A, Di MENZA C, BRUGERE-PICOUX J, BRUGERE H, CHATELAIN J AND BUVET R. (1992) Electroanalytical characterization of Alzheimer's disease and ovine spongiform encephalopathy by repeated cyclic voltametry at a capillary graphite paste electrode. Bioelectrochemistry and Bioenergetics *28*, 127-147.

BENNETT A D, BIRKETT C R AND BOSTOCK C J. (1992) Molecular biology of scrapie-like agents. Rev. sci. tech. Off. int. Epiz. *11*, 569-603.

BLISARD K S, DAVIS L E, HARRINGTON M G, LOVELL J K, KORNFELD M AND BERGER M L. (1990) Pre-mortem diagnosis of Creutzfeldt-Jakob disease by detection of abnormal cerebrospinal fluid proteins. J. Neurol. Sci. *99*, 75-81.

BRUCE M, CHREE A, McCONNELL I, FOSTER J, PEARSON G AND FRASER H. (1994) Transmission of bovine spongiform encephalopathy and scrapie to mice: strain variation and the species barrier. Phil. Trans. Roy. Soc. Series B *343*, 405-411.

COLLINGE J, WHITTINGTON M A, SIDLE K C L, SMITH C J, PALMER M S, CLARKE A R AND JEFFREYS J G R. (1994) Prion protein is necessary for normal synaptic function. Nature *370*, 295-297.

KELLINGS K, MEYER N, MIRENDA C, PRUSINER S B AND RIESNER D. (1993). Analysis of nucleic acids in purified scrapie prion preparations. Arch. Virol. *7*, 215-225.

KIMBERLIN R H. (1990) Scrapie and possible relationships with viroids. Semin. Virol. *1*, 153-162.

KOCISKO D A, COME J H, PRIOLA S A, CHESBORO B, RAYMOND G J, LANSBURY P T AND CAUGHEY B. (1994) Cell-free formation of protease-resistant prion protein. Nature *370*, 471-474.

ÖZEL M AND DIRINGER H. (1994) Small virus-like structure in fractions from scrapie hamster brain. Lancet *343*, 894-895.

PRUSINER S B. (1993) Genetic and infectious prion diseases. Arch. Virol. *50*, 1129-1153.

ROHWER R G. (1991) The scrapie agent: "A virus by any other name". In: Current Topics in Microbiology and Immunology *172*, 195-232.

SCHREUDER B E C. (1994) BSE agent hypotheses. Livestock Production Science. Special Issue. *38*, 23-33.

SCOTT M, FOSTER D, MIRENDA C, SERBAN D, COUFAL F, WÄLCHLI M, TORCHIA M, GROTH D, CARLSON G, DeARMOND S J, WESTAWAY D AND PRUSINER S B. (1989) Transgenic mice expressing hamster prion protein produce species-specific scrapie infectivity and amyloid plaques. Cell *59*, 847-857.

STAHL N, BALDWIN M A, TEPLOW D B, HOOD L, GIBSON B W, BURLINGAME A L AND PRUSINER S B. (1993) Structural studies of the scrapie prion protein using mass spectrometry and amino acid sequencing. Biochemistry *32*, 1991-2002.

WEISSMANN C. (1991) A "Unified Theory" of prion propagation. Nature *352*, 679-683.

WILLS P R. (1991) Prion diseases and the frame-shifting hypothesis. N.Z. Vet. J. *39*, 41-45.

YUN M, WU W, HOOD L AND HARRINGTON M. (1992) Human cerebrospinal fluid protein database: Edition 1992. Electrophoresis *13*, 1002-1013.

ADDENDUM TO CHAPTER 6

SOME ALTERNATIVE HYPOTHESES ON THE
AETIOLOGY OF TRANSMISSIBLE
SPONGIFORM ENCEPHALOPATHIES

6.10 *Introduction*

The preceding chapters recount current knowledge
of TSE, including the results of recent research,
much of which is generally accepted but some
disputed. For example, we still do not understand
TSE agent structure, in particular the nature of its
genome and how it replicates as exemplified by the
prion, virino and virus hypotheses, the normal
function of PrP or the exact means of transmission
of infection. Additional to these major hypotheses
are a number of others, which require mention to
indicate the widely ranging concepts of agent
structure and hypotheses concerning the origin and
cause of BSE and other recently recognised TSEs of
animals.

Intestinal fluid dependent organisms (IFDO)

A novel replicating agent (IFDO), which shares
some characteristics with CJD agent, has been
isolated from human ileal fluid. This agent may be
an intestinal commensal but is remarkably resistant
to inactivation by steam at 134°C, sodium
hydroxide, aldehyde fixatives, trypsin, Proteinase K
and ionising radiation. IFDOs can pass filters with a
pore diameter of 10nm. Unlike scrapie however,
IFDOs are inactivated by ethidium bromide, zinc
nitrate, ribonuclease, EDTA and hydroxylamine in
the presence of Sarkosyl. The replicating agent may
be formed by crystallisation from constituents of the
culture medium and not by a biological process.
Studies to isolate IFDO from normal and diseased
sheep (scrapie) and cattle (BSE) brain were
inconclusive. Unpublished findings have identified
that lipoprotein and other substances are needed for
IFDO replication. However, when IFDOs are
incubated with these substances they are no longer
inactivated by zinc nitrate and are highly resistant to
ribonuclease. The particles, in this form, resemble
prions. Whereas this work does not advance our
knowledge of TSE agents in any significant way it
suggests that there is a class of agents with some
similar properties to prions.

Nucleation and crystallisation

Several hypotheses have been put forward to
suggest that some form of nucleation or *in vivo*
crystallisation of PrP^{Sc} in TSEs is responsible for
disease. These may not be easily distinguished from
the conformational templating mechanism (see para
6.7) and might best be regarded as a variant of the
prion hypothesis. A similar transformation of
β-amyloid precursor protein is proposed in
Alzheimer's disease and other amyloidoses.
However, though amyloid plaques which might be
formed by nucleation are present in some TSEs,
they have not been found in others.

Molecular chaperones

A theory has been developed that prions could be
molecular chaperones (see glossary) that are
required for their own assembly. This theory has
been deduced from an analysis of protein folding
and the consequences explored by computer
simulation. Thus, a protein could behave as a new
kind of informational molecule mimicking an
infectious process. Whether 'replication' is a
biological or 'chemical' phenomenon remains to be
seen, but there do seem potentially to be some
similarities.

ssDNA

Mention has already been made (see para 6.8) that
using unconventional methods, one worker has
suggested a single-stranded DNA with a unique
palindromic nucleotide sequence is the agent
genome, or part of it. Other workers have
discounted this hypothesis. Nevertheless, work is in
hand to independently investigate this using
identical methods. No results are yet available. It is
suggested that the agent is a 'nemavirus' which can
be seen in thin sections by electron microscopy. The
nemavirus is claimed to have three layers: an outer
coat of protease-sensitive material, a central layer
comprising ssDNA and an inner core of PrP^{Sc}. This
hypothetical structure is so far unsubstantiated
though structures equated with 'nemavirus' or
tubulofilamentous bodies are seen uniquely in
electron micrographs of brain tissue in scrapie-like
diseases.

Green cluster nutrients and BSE

It has been claimed that chronic deficiency of green cluster nutrients, and in particular loss of α-linolenic acid (the omega 3 precursor for docosahexaenoic acid needed for brain growth) and linoleic acid, could have increased the susceptibility of cattle to BSE. The hypothesis is based on clinical, biochemical studies in healthy captive wild ruminants in a zoo compared with those in the wild. It is also based on assumed changes in the grazing and feeding of sheep and cattle eg a move from vegetable protein (soya) feeding of cattle to meat and bone meal (animal protein) feeding. These latter changes have not been substantiated by epidemiological studies of BSE, and there is no evidence to show that cattle are in fact deficient in these fatty acids.

Use of high nitrogen fertilisers and BSE

It has been claimed that use of high nitrogen fertilisers is a factor in inducing BSE. This specific association is not a common factor for BSE occurrence and indeed beef cattle kept entirely on grass and conserved products appear not to be at risk from BSE despite nitrogen fertiliser application. Variations on this theme have also been proposed eg the fundamental cause of BSE is the consumption of excessive quantities of protein that stimulates the release of somatotrophin and encourages gluconeogenesis. However, similar levels of protein feeding of cattle are used elsewhere in the world, notably in mainland Europe and North America, where BSE either does not occur, or is at a very low incidence. Furthermore, there is no identifiable change in protein feeding of cattle that is temporally related to the emergence of BSE in 1985/86.

Organophosphorus compounds (OPC)

Use of OPCs as insecticides, particularly during the campaign to eradicate warble fly, has been claimed either to cause BSE or render cows susceptible to BSE. The original epidemiological investigation considered any possible association between the use of agricultural chemicals, including OP insecticides,

and the occurrence of BSE. None was found. The lesions of delayed neurotoxicity induced by OPC are clearly distinguishable from those in BSE. Many other countries without BSE use OPCs on cattle and contrariwise. Guernsey, on which island OPCs are not significantly used, does have BSE. Again there is no explanation for the temporal occurrence of BSE by the OPC hypothesis.

A bacterial hypothesis

Another hypothesis suggests the agent causing TSEs is a bacterium. The basis for this is the finding of spiroplasma-like inclusions in brain tissue of biopsies or autopsy brains from patients with CJD, and immunological cross-reactivity between spiroplasma broth culture and PrP^{sc}. This unusual theory is not supported by the available evidence.

Neuronal cell membrane hypothesis

A recent publication reporting results of much earlier radiation experiments shows the agent is effectively transparent to germicidal ultraviolet radiation, and claims that replication cannot involve coding by a nucleic acid, nor can the informational-conveying component be protein. The studies support an earlier hypothesis that the agent is a fragment of neuronal cell membrane.

6.11 Comments on alternative hypotheses

Before any of these hypotheses can be considered viable and justifiable to test, the basis for them should be published in peer-reviewed scientific journals and the work leading to their evolution be verified independently. We do not perceive that there is currently any justification for extending any of the above studies within the current TSE research programme. For the present, it is sufficient to recognise that there are two main hypotheses (prion hypothesis and virino hypothesis), with a large number of variants powerfully supported by individuals. The main differences between them and problems for each have changed little since Kimberlin questioned and wrote on 'scrapie agent: prions or virinos?' in 1982.

Printed in the United Kingdom for HMSO
Dd 0300148   C9   1/95   65536   O/N 312444   01/31886

Reading list

ALPER T. (1993) The scrapie enigma: insights from radiation experiments. Radiat. Res. *135*, 283-292.

ARANDA-ANZALDO A. (1992) Possible cell-free prion replication. Med. Hypotheses *38*, 249-251.

BASTIAN F O. (1993) Bovine spongiform encephalopathy: relationship to human disease and nature of the agent. Am. Soc. Microbiol. *59*, 235-240.

BURDON D W. (1989) A novel replicating agent isolated from the human intestinal tract having characteristics shared with Creutzfeldt-Jakob and related agents. J. Med. Microbiol. *29*, 145-157.

COME J H, FRASER P E AND LANSBURY P T Jr. (1993) A kinetic model for amyloid formation in the prion diseases: importance of seeding. Proc. Natl. Acad. Sci. USA *90*, 5959-5963.

CRAWFORD M A, BUDOWSKI P, DRURY P, GHERBREMESKEL K, HARBIGE L, LEIGHFIELD M, PHYLACTOS A AND

WILLIAMS G. (1991) The nutritional contribution to bovine spongiform encephalopathy. Nutr. Health *7*, 61-68.

DeARMOND S J. (1993) Alzheimer's disease and Creutzfeldt-Jakob disease: overlap of pathogenic mechanisms. Curr. Opin. Neurol. *6*, 872-881.

DIRINGER H. (1992) Hidden amyloidoses. Exp. Clin. Immunogenet. *9*, 212-229.

GAJDUSEK D C. (1994) Spontaneous generation of infectious nucleating amyloids in the transmissible and non-transmissible cerebral amyloidoses. Molec. Neurobiol. *8*, 1-13.

JARRETT J T AND LANSBURY P T Jr. (1993) Seeding "one-dimensional crystallization" of amyloid: a pathogenic mechanism in Alzheimer's disease and scrapie? Cell *73*, 1055-1058.

KIMBERLIN R H. (1982) Scrapie agents: prions or virinos? Nature *297*, 107-108.

LIAUTARD J P. (1993) Prions and molecular chaperones. Arch. Virol. *7*, 227-243.

NARANG H K. (1993) Evidence that scrapie-associated tubulofilamentous particles contain a single-stranded DNA. Intervirology *36* (1), 1-10.

PRIOLA S A, CAUGHEY B, RACE R E AND CHESEBRO B. (1994) Heterologous PrP molecules interfere with accumulation of protease-resistant PrP in scrapie-infected murine neuroblastoma cells. J. Virol. *68*, 4873-4878.

PURDEY M. (1992) Mad cows and warble flies: a link between BSE and organophosphates. The Ecologist *22*, 52-57.

PURDEY M. (1994) Are organosphosphate pesticides involved in the causation of bovine spongiform encephalopathy (BSE)? Hypothesis based on a literature review and limited trials on BSE cattle. J. Nutr. Med. *4*, 43-82.

Recent Research and Some Specific Questions

7.1 *Introduction*

One of the main functions of the SEAC is to give views on the needs and priorities for research into the transmissible spongiform encephalopathies; especially that research which is crucial to enable sound advice to be given on matters concerning public health and animal health, particularly for animals reared for the production of human food. The first interim report addressed these questions and the second reported the response of MAFF, DoH, AFRC, MRC, other funding bodies and researchers to the recommendations. Results from some of the initial experiments, including some of the infectivity studies involving lengthy incubation periods in rodents, have now come to fruition and others are well advanced, and we have been able to include some results in this report. The spongiform encephalopathies form a very difficult field for research because the fundamental nature of the disease is only partly understood, most experiments take a long time to do, results are slow to come in and funds are liable to run out before they are complete. It is therefore not harshly critical to say that in spite of many successes important questions remain unanswered. In our view research is most likely to be productive and relevant if it starts with a clear hypothesis or aims to answer a specific question. We therefore give below some questions which might help the planning of future research.

7.2 *Recent research*

In recent years important new findings, such as the occurrence of mutations in *PrP* gene, have been made. These have led to a much fuller understanding of pedigrees of familial CJD and GSS. In sheep, resistance and susceptibility to natural and experimental scrapie seems to be largely due to variation in the *PrP* gene. As so often in science these advances depended on work done entirely independently, namely the development of the polymerase chain reaction (PCR), using Taq polymerase, to amplify specific regions of DNA. If infectivity turned out to be associated with specific nucleic acid then PCR would provide a rapid and specific diagnostic method. Instead we have to use the relatively non-specific methods for PrP^{Sc} detection. Bioassay is much more sensitive but quite impractical for field use. A test for infectivity, other than bioassay, is therefore an important research goal. It is thus very important to continue research aimed at detecting a nucleic acid agent genome, or some other molecular entity which adequately explains such phenomena as mutation and strain types. This is likely to arise as a by-product of basic studies by research workers who have a degree of good fortune and the ability to recognise the key piece of a jigsaw when it presents itself.

Research has also been affected by another relatively new technology, mammalian transgenics. Mice have been produced with normal hamster *PrP* genes, with additional normal or mutant human *PrP* genes, with chimaeric mouse/hamster genes or with deleted *PrP* genes. It is also possible to generate mice without mouse *PrP* genes but with normal cattle, sheep or human *PrP* genes instead. These have given valuable information on the importance of *PrP*. These results offer the hope of improved methods of testing for infectivity of SEs, but more basic knowledge and practical testing are required.

We need to know how many copies of which genes will increase sensitivity for specific agents. Other genes could be involved and might need to be identified and inserted as well as *PrP*. Environmental factors and route of inoculation would also need to be optimized.

Work has also been undertaken on the non-coding strand of the *PrP* gene and its hypothetical product 'Anti-PrP', for which there is some evidence since its mRNA has been detected in more than one species. The most recent research suggests, however, that this may arise from another gene since it has also been detected in mice in which the *PrP* gene has been deleted. Also, both old and new research (Westaway *et al* 1994) has suggested that 'antisense PrP RNAs are not derived from the *PrP* gene locus but represent artifactual cross-hybridisation, possibly mediated by G + C-rich sequences within the N-terminus of the *PrP* gene open reading frame'. Thus genetic studies need to be continued in the natural hosts of TSEs, especially humans, sheep and perhaps captive wild ruminants and cats. It could also be imperative to study animals such as pigs, chickens and also certain ruminants and FELIDAE in zoos that have been fed BSE-infected feed and have remained unaffected - pathological studies, assays for infectivity and PrP, and sequencing of *PrP* could begin to explain this.

The epidemiology of natural sheep scrapie is poorly understood and would benefit from the application of *PrP* genotypes in defined populations for which a full breeding history is available and where flock owners are open about the existence of disease. This could benefit animal health. It has been postulated that in geographic, familial clusters of CJD in Slovakia, where susceptibility is clearly related to *PrP* mutations, exposure to an exogenous pathogenic agent may also be necessary for disease to result. Information is meagre but if the hypothesis were to be correct, even in very rare circumstances, it could provide information of value in understanding the disease and its prevention.

The BSE epidemic in Great Britain is declining and the disease may be eradicated from the UK by the control measures already in place. However, we note the substantial proportion (15%) of suspect cases which are unconfirmed by subsequent laboratory examination. The number of

unconfirmed cases of BSE is currently high in certain groups, including young and old age classes, and is costly to investigate and compensate. It is important to investigate negative cases, both to discover what they are due to and to reduce their proportion by devising means of improved diagnosis in the live animal *eg* by improved clinical observation or ancillary tests. It should also be a target to diagnose these 'negative' cases specifically before or after death - perhaps new metabolic diseases could be identified and treated, to the benefit of animal health. The definitive clinical signs of BSE are under study and have already revealed changes in rumination and heart rate that are associated with the diseased state and such work should be extended.

The BSE epidemic has highlighted our lack of understanding of the factors involved in maternal transmission. It is unlikely that of all mammals, only the placenta of sheep is able to harbour the agent. There is no obvious organised nervous or lymphoid tissue in the placenta so in which cells is the agent present? Far too little research has been conducted in this area, for lack of a convenient model. New methods are needed, perhaps using mice transgenic for the ovine and bovine *PrP* gene.

Studies on tissue infectivity and susceptibility are very important; not least, for example, to determine if scrapie 'resistant' (pApA) Cheviot sheep harbour infection, act as carriers, and transmit infection to other sheep. What is needed is a cell culture system that could rapidly replicate agent and allow its early detection, and thus replace the use of animals. We welcome continued efforts to develop such cell lines using either transgenic animal tissues or those from 'resistant' and 'susceptible' sheep.

The origin of BSE is as yet unconfirmed, although it has been postulated that it might have come from sheep scrapie or from a sub-clinical form of BSE in cattle. Experiments to determine whether scrapie can transmit orally to cattle have been conducted in the USA, but none has been attempted in Britain. This is surprising, considering the long existence of scrapie in the country. More studies of scrapie strains from sheep and goat isolates might show whether strains of the BSE agent type infect sheep naturally. Further experiments might suggest the origin of BSE (*ie* whether BSE came from sheep with scrapie, or from cattle), the nature of the sheep/cattle species barrier, and possible future hazards and control measures.

7.3 Some specific questions

The nature of the agent(s)

This report has considered some possible and some unlikely hypotheses above (see paras 6.10 and 6.11) but none answers satisfactorily all the questions raised by present knowledge, such as:-

▲ Why is disease-specific PrP central to the disease process?

▲ If the host of origin (the *PrP* gene) influences the species barrier why does it not always influence the virulence for inbred mice, manifested as 'strain variation'?

▲ Why is infectivity so stable to heat and other physical and chemical treatments?

▲ Given that there is a genetic component of the agent, why has no characteristic nucleic acid been found?

▲ In those cases of familial human TSEs which are strongly associated with pathogenic *PrP* gene mutations, where does the transmissible agent come from? Is it simply the protein coded for by the gene?

The pathological changes

▲ What is the structure of PrP^c and how is it changed into PrP^{Sc}? A comparative crystallographic analysis of both forms of the protein would be one way to address this question experimentally.

▲ If the change from PrP^c to PrP^{Sc} is purely conformational, *ie* does not involve covalent linkages, can the change be propagated *in vitro?*

▲ Can PrP^{Sc} convert PrP^c to PrP^{Sc} if they are mixed in appropriate conditions?

▲ What initiates this change and how can it be detected?

▲ Can we specify the three dimensional configuration in the molecule or that part of it which changes in disease? Is there a difference in this configuration in different strains of, say, scrapie?

▲ Can native PrP^{Sc}, especially with pathogenic sequences, induce disease?

▲ What are the normal sites of PrP^c? This needs research well 'tuned-in' to current investigations of the protein-protein interactions and mode of action of molecular chaperones that underlie the functional and conformational changes that occur in, for example, blood clotting, embryo development and oncogenesis. Is there any way of reducing PrP^{Sc} accumulation or minimising its pathological effect?

▲ By what mechanism does over expression of wild-type *PrP* gene cause necrotising myopathy and polyneuropathy in mice?

Transmission

▲ Under conditions of normal husbandry, can BSE be transmitted to cattle other than by feed?

▲ Are the cases of sporadic CJD that occur in patients with a higher occupational exposure to BSE:

- clinically different from CJD cases in other occupational groups?

- associated with agent of the BSE strain type?

▲ By what mechanisms does infection transmit between greater kudu in captivity?

▲ In one experimental study transgenic mice overexpressing a *PrP* mutant (equivalent to GSS codon 102) gene have developed apparently spontaneous spongiform encephalopathy which is apparently transmissible to further mice (see para 6.12). However, since no PrP^{Sc} was found in these mice the result is dubious. Therefore a crucial experiment will be to repeat this study independently to determine whether a transmissible agent has been generated. A successful transmission would give support to the prion hypothesis.

Control of BSE epidemic

▲ Will the epidemic continue to decline according to the present epidemic model?

▲ Is the BSE strain type associated with recent cases the same as that found with earlier cases?

▲ What are the causes of the nervous diseases of the cattle which present clinically like BSE?

▲ Does the occurrence of BSE in other countries parallel the UK experience or provide any new clues on the epidemiology and control of BSE?

Important applied questions

▲ Will any further species become affected?

▲ What is the present frequency and distribution of scrapie in various sheep-rearing countries and what strains are circulating in different sheep and goat populations?

▲ Can it be shown that there is a satisfactory way of inactivating TSE infectivity in the rendering industry?

▲ Are there effective non-destructive ways of disinfecting hospital equipment and instruments contaminated with TSE agents?

7.4 Research programmes

These problems can only be tackled effectively by multidisciplinary research by teams whose members have common interests and experiments but differing expertise and background knowledge.

It is clear that exchange of reagents has facilitated progress in many laboratories *eg* characterised strains of scrapie, anti-PrP sera and cell lines. There is room for more of these collaborative activities.

A really convenient experimental animal host in which to test pathogenicity for man - perhaps a transgenic mouse strain - is badly needed, as is a productive *in vitro* model of both neural and other cell types.

7.5 CONCLUDING REMARKS - some implications for research

It is disappointing, but not surprising that the study of PrP has not yet led to an *in vivo* diagnostic test, or to ideas for preventing or reversing the progress of pathological changes. The basic reason is, we believe, the intrinsic difficulty of the scientific questions and the experimental methods used. Development of more convenient and 'quicker' (*ie* enable detection of infectivity in a short time span) *in vitro* models could accelerate progress. We hope this area of research will be further developed.

We note that tests to detect specific biochemical abnormalities may yet become available for clinicians. However, we are afraid those being studied at present may not be sensitive enough to detect human cases soon enough for therapeutic intervention or in animals as a support to epidemiological study or possible culling. One exception would be detection of *PrP* gene mutations in healthy family members of patients which, if a suitable treatment became available, could perhaps delay the onset or prevent disease occurrence.

The experiments on the reduction of infectivity by rendering have provided useful confirmation of the epidemiological evidence that the epidemic was able to start because rendering practices were changed. However, the origin of the infection in cattle, whether from sheep scrapie or from an endemic infection of cattle, is not certain. It is difficult to conceive of a design for a further rendering experiment that would provide scientifically convincing evidence to guarantee the safety of meat and bone meal in regard to TSE agents, and therefore justify the re-introduction of such feed into ruminant rations. Therefore on scientific grounds it may be necessary to maintain a ruminant feed ban indefinitely to ensure protection of ruminant species from TSE agents via feed.

The BSE epidemic has had serious effects on both animal health and the agricultural industry. It is now clear that the incidence has reached a peak and is declining, we believe because of the control measures instituted in the late 1980s. However, it would be unwise to forecast exactly how the epidemic will decline. We cannot be certain that all the cases of BSE in animals 'born after the ban' were infected by contaminated feed that was still in the pipeline. There is still no evidence of significant transmission from dam to offspring, but this could occur even now and extend the epidemic albeit at lower levels unless accompanied by horizontal transmission. Comprehensive and critical monitoring of the epidemic must be maintained.

Recent data provided to MAFF by the industry indicate that very little infectivity probably entered the human food chain after November 1989, the date when all specified bovine offals were statutorily removed from the human food chains. There is no evidence that contaminated food consumed before that date has induced a rise in CJD or related disease of man. In view of the long incubation period of kuru (a disease induced by eating contaminated human tissues), continued observation of CJD is needed for several years yet - perhaps a decade or two in case such a rise, however unlikely, occurs later.

The cases of CJD induced by contaminated surgical instruments, transplants, and by injection of pituitary-derived hormones, occurred because basic information about CJD was not applied soon enough or effectively enough. However, cases resulting from these causes will decline eventually as action has been taken to prevent the repetition of such incidents.

In the case of the much larger epidemic of BSE, we were fortunate that the causative strain was not readily transmitted between cattle under natural farming conditions. There was a great deal of information about scrapie, which provided a sound basis for devising control measures. However, it was important that epidemiological data were quickly and carefully gathered to identify the source of infection. Now that the epidemic is visibly under control it is important that all the control measures (including those to protect non-ruminants) are stringently enforced for as long as is necessary to eliminate the epidemic.

Reading list

GRANGER J AND MADDEN D. (1993) The polymerase chain reaction: turning needles into haystacks. Biologist *40*, 197-200.

GOLDGABER D. (1991) Anticipating the anti-prion protein? Scientific correspondence. Nature *351*, 106.

HEWINSON R G, LOWINGS J P, DAWSON M D AND WOODWARD M J. (1991) Anti-prions and other agents. Scientific correspondence. Nature *352*, 291.

MOSER M, OESCH B AND BÜELER H. (1993) An anti-prion protein? Nature *362*, 213-214.

PRUSINER S B, SCOTT M, FOSTER D, PAN K M, GROTH D, MIRENDA C, TORCHIA, M, YANG S.L, SERBAN D, CARLSON G A, HOPPE P C, WESTAWAY D AND DeARMOND S J. (1990) Transgenetic studies implicate interactions between homologous PrP isoforms in scrapie prion replication. Cell *63*, 673-686.

SCOTT M, GROTH D, FOSTER D, TORCHIA M, YANG S L, DeARMOND S J AND PRUSINER S B. (1993) Propagation of prions with artificial properties in transgenic mice expressing chimeric *PrP* genes. Cell *73*, 979-988.

WESTAWAY D, COOPER C, TURNER S, D A COSTA M, CARLSON G A AND PRUSINER S B. (1994) Structure and polymorphism of the mouse prion protein gene. Proc. Natl. Acad. Sci. *91*, 6418-6422.

Acknowledgements

A large number of people have contributed to the production of this report, too many to mention individually. However, we wish to thank particularly staff at

the Central Veterinary Laboratory Weybridge;

the Institute for Animal Health, BBSRC/MRC Neuropathogenesis Unit in Edinburgh;

the Medical Research Council;

National Institutes of Health, National Institute of Neurological Disorders and Stroke, Laboratory of Central Nervous System Studies, Bethesda, Maryland and the Laboratory of Persistent Viral Diseases, Rocky Mountain Laboratories, Hamilton, Montana, USA;

the Ministry of Agriculture, Fisheries and Food (MAFF), Animal Health Veterinary Group at Tolworth and the Department of Health, CJD Surveillance Unit in Edinburgh for provision of data and/or scrutiny of particular chapters of the report.

In particular we thank the following individuals for critical comments and advice on the draft report:

Professor R M Barlow
Professor J Brockes
Dr P Brown
Dr M Bruce
Dr B W Chesebro
Dr S Gore
Mr M T Haddon
Mr B Harris
Dr J Hope
Dr N Hunter
Professor P Jordan
Professor P Lowry
Dr D Matthews
Mr G A H Wells
Mr J W Wilesmith

We thank also Mrs E M Davies for typing the script, Mrs W Bolton for secretarial assistance, Mrs C Humphries, Mrs Y I Spencer (CVL) and Dr D Matthews for preparing some of the figures and Mrs S Townsend and other staff of the MAFF, Animal Health (Disease Control) Division for organising publication via Mr R Myers of MAFF Publicity Branch Tolworth, and HMSO, who collectively gave constructive advice on presentational aspects.

Glossary of Abbreviations and Scientific Terms

'A' group scrapie strains: Scrapie strains which have a shorter incubation when inoculated into *Sip* sAsA sheep than in *Sip* pApA sheep. Most strains belong to this group. See: 'C' group scrapie strains.

ACDP: Advisory Committee on Dangerous Pathogens: advises the Health and Safety Commission, the Health and Safety Executive and Health and Agriculture Ministers as required on all aspects of hazards and risks to workers and others from exposure to pathogens.

AFRC: Agricultural and Food Research Council (see also BBSRC).

Agent: Term being used to describe the infectious micro-organisms responsible for the spongiform encephalopathies: not yet clearly identified or isolated: could be an atypical virus, a specific nucleic acid complexed with a host derived protein ('virino') or only protein ('prion').

Allele: The component of a gene derived from one parent and contributing hereditary information from that parent.

Amyloid: A fibrillar protein found in various pathological states and showing characteristic apple green birefringence when stained with Congo red.

APHIS: Animal and Plant Health Inspection Service (USDA).

ARIA: Acetylcholine receptor inducing activity.

Astroglia: Also known as astrocytes - supporting cells to neurons in the CNS. In the CNS astrocytes are activated in scrapie-like diseases, a condition known as astrogliosis.

Ataxia: Inability to co-ordinate voluntary movement.

Autosomal dominant: A gene forming part of a chromosome that is not a sex chromosome, which produces the same character when it is present in single dose as when present in double dose (*ie* when the two alleles are identical).

BBSRC: Biotechnology and Biological Sciences Research Council (Established in and incorporating the AFRC on 1 April 1994).

bp: Base pair of nucleotides of DNA.

BSE: Bovine spongiform encephalopathy, the new spongiform encephalopathy in British and other cattle.

'C' group scrapie strains: Scrapie strains which have a longer incubation when inoculated into *Sip* sAsA sheep than in *Sip* pApA sheep. Only one strain CH1641, has so far been allocated to the 'C' group.

Caudal: Concerning or towards the tail.

CCR: Consultative Committee on Research (1st Tyrrell Committee).

cDNA: Complementary DNA copied from RNA.

CDSC: Communicable Disease Surveillance Centre: responsible for monitoring human infectious diseases in England and Wales.

CD(S)U: Communicable Disease (Scotland) Unit.

Challenge: The experimental event which aims to establish infection in the host.

CJD: Creutzfeldt-Jakob disease, a human spongiform encephalopathy.

Codon: A triplet of bases in a nucleic acid sequence which determines a particular amino acid in protein synthesis.

CNS: Central nervous system.

Congophilic: Having an affinity for the dye (stain) Congo red which stains amyloid.

Contagious: Transmitted by direct contact.

CSF: Cerebrospinal fluid, the fluid that bathes the brain and spinal cord.

CSM: Committee on Safety of Medicines.

CVL: Central Veterinary Laboratory, an agency of MAFF, responsible for co-ordinating the surveillance of and investigation of animal diseases.

CWD: Chronic wasting disease of mule deer, Rocky Mountain elk and a few other CERVIDAE, but only in North America.

Da: Dalton - 'unit' of molecular weight.

DES: Department of Education and Science.

DoH: Department of Health.

Dominant: See autosomal dominant and recessive gene.

Downer cows: Refers to the clinical manifestation of being unable to rise. It is a common occurrence, usually around parturition, and can result from a variety of causes. The main clinical sign is an inability to stand. It is conceivable that a proportion of cases are due to infection with the BSE agent even though BSE has never been identified in the US.

DNA: Deoxyribonucleic acid.

EC: European Commission.

EEG: Electroencephalogram.

EM: Electron microscopy.

Episome: A genetically active particle able to exist and multiply independently or integrated into a chromosome.

EU: European Union.

Exposure: The natural event which initiates infection in the host.

F$_1$ hybrid: The first cross of two separate line-bred (established) strains.

Fibril: see SAF.

FFI: Fatal familial insomnia.

FSE: Feline spongiform encephalopathy.

Genes and gene function: The major function of a gene is to code for the production of proteins. Genes comprise variable nucleotide sequences of deoxyribonucleic acid (DNA) which occur in chromosomes in the cell nucleus. DNA is a polymer of nucleotides, each comprising a base, a sugar and a phosphate molecule. The sequence of four bases (adenine, guanine, cytosine and thymine) in the polynucleotide chain constitutes the code to produce particular amino acids via ribonucleic acid (RNA), a process called transcription. RNA then translates the message in the cell cytoplasm where amino acids are assembled to form proteins. At some sites within a gene two alternative nucleotides may exist. Such genes are called polymorphic and may result in different phenotypes if the altered code results in the translation of a different amino acid.

Genotype: The genetic constitution (allelic make-up) of an organism.

GB: Great Britain.

GFAP: Glial fibrillar acid protein, a molecular marker for astrocytes.

Glycosylated: Having linkage with a glycosyl (carbohydrate) group.

GPI: Glycophosphatidylinositol.

GSS: Gerstmann-Sträussler-Scheinker disease, a rare familial form of CJD, now known to be associated with mutations in the *PrP* gene.

HaB: Hamster brain.

Heterodimer: In the context of PrP^{Sc} synthesis, hypothesised to be an intermediate protein duplex consisting of two molecules (dimer), one of PrP^c and one of PrP^{Sc} which produces two new molecules of PrP^{Sc}.

Heterozygous: Having different alleles in the two corresponding loci (positions) of a pair of chromosomes.

hGH: Human growth hormone - at one time made from pituitaries from human cadavers rarely and inadvertently contaminated with CJD agent, and now known to have transmitted CJD to a small number of those treated with hGH for short stature.

Home-bred: Animals which reside on the farm on which they were born.

Homozygous: Having identical alleles in the two corresponding loci (positions) of a pair of chromosomes.

hPG: Human pituitary-derived gonadotrophin (see also hGH above).

HPLC: High performance liquid chromatography.

Iatrogenic transmission: Accidental transmission; literally - 'born of doctors' *ie* a result of medical or veterinary procedures.

IAH: Institute for Animal Health.

i/c: Intracerebral.

ID$_{50}$: Infectious dose required to kill 50% of the challenged animals.

IEF: Isoelectric focusing.

IFDO: Intestinal fluid dependent organism.

Immunoblot (Western blot): Biological materials are separated in an electric field (electrophoresis) and transferred to a sheet on which they can be stained with a specific antisera. This shows that certain sized protein molecules combine with the antibody used.

Infectious: Caused by a micro-organism.

IP: Incubation period.

kb: kilobase pair = one thousand base pairs.

kDa: kiloDalton = one thousand 'units' of molecular weight.

Lateral (horizontal) transmission: Transmission between related or unrelated individuals other than by genetic or maternal transmission (qv).

LR: Lymphoreticular.

LRS: Lymphoreticular system.

Lysosome: An intracellular organelle containing enzymes which play a role in intracellular digestion.

MAFF: Ministry of Agriculture, Fisheries and Food.

Maternal transmission: Transmission from dam to offspring *in utero* or in the immediate *post partum* period.

MBM: Meat and bone meal.

Microglia: Supporting phagocytic cells in the central nervous system which are activated during inflammation.

Molecular chaperones: Fundamental cellular proteins that interact with newly formed proteins to ensure they take up the correct structure. They often increase in response to 'stress'.

moi: Multiplicity of infection.

M$_r$: Molecular ratio - roughly equivalent to molecular weight.

MRC: Medical Research Council.

mRNA: Messenger RNA - nucleic acid carrying instructions from DNA (the gene) for making specific proteins.

Myristylated: Containing myristic (tetradecanoic) acid.

Natural transmission: Transmission by any method other than deliberate or accidental exposure or challenge.

Nucleotide: A compound of a nucleoside and phosphoric acid which forms the principal constituent of nucleic acid.

Neurite: Appendage (process) of a nerve cell; composed of multiple dendrites and a single axon which receive or transmit nervous impulses.

Neuron: Nerve cell.

Neuropil: CNS grey matter comprising the processes of neurons.

NGF: Nerve growth factor.

NIBSC: National Institute for Biological Standards and Control.

NPU: Neuropathogenesis Unit of the Institute for Animal Health BBSRC/MRC; research unit working on spongiform encephalopathies.

Occupational exposure: The initiation of a human infection in the course of the patient's occupation.

OPCs: Organophosphorus compounds.

PAGE: *Poly*acrylamide *g*el *e*lectrophoresis.

Parenteral: Administered by any way other than through the mouth.

PC: Phaeochromocytoma cell line.

PCR: Polymerase chain reaction.

Peripheral route: The initiation of infection *via* any route other than via the central nervous system *eg* intravenous, subcutaneous or intraperitoneal inoculation.

Phenotype: The characteristics manifested by an organism.

PI: Phosphatidylinositol.

PIPLC: Phosphatidylinositol-specific phospholipase C.

Polymorphism: Structural variation in a gene, which may or may not code for different amino acids at the same site.

Proteinase K: A powerful enzyme for digesting proteins.

PrP: The normal form PrP is a host-coded protein that becomes modified and partially protease resistant in infected tissue and accumulates around CNS lesions in transmissible spongiform encephalopathies. The protease resistant form PrP^{Sc} is a major component of SAF.

***PrP* gene:** A widely conserved host gene coding for PrP^{C}.

PrP^{C}: PrP^{Cellular} the normal cellular isoform of PrP.

PrP^{Sc}: PrP^{Scrapie} the abnormal disease-specific isoform of PrP derived post-translationally from PrP^{C}.

psi: Pounds per square inch.

Recessive gene: A gene which usually has no effect on the phenotype unless present in a double dose (*ie* when both alleles are the same).

Rendering: Processing offal and discarded animal carcases to make, *inter alia,* meat and bone meal for animal feed.

RFLP: *R*estriction *F*ragment. A portion of a gene of a defined length created by treatment of DNA with specific restriction endonuclease enzymes - *L*ength *P*olymorphism means variability in the length from one individual to another.

Rida: The Icelandic name for scrapie.

Rida area: The geographically defined area of Iceland where rida originally established itself.

RNA: Ribonucleic acid.

Rostral: Concerning or towards the head (literally the beak).

RVC: Royal Veterinary College, London.

SAF: Scrapie associated fibrils; abnormal structures detected by electron microscopy of extracts of brains of spongiform encephalopathy cases. Composed of modified PrP.

sA/pA and s^{7}/p^{7}: Represent the alleles of *Sip* and *Sinc* genes encoding for short (s) and prolonged (p) incubation periods of scrapie in sheep and mice respectively.

SBO: Specified bovine offals comprising brain, spinal cord, thymus, tonsil, spleen and intestine (from duodenum to rectum inclusive) from cattle over 6 months old - and thymus and intestine from cattle of any age.

Scrapie: A spongiform encephlopathy of sheep. Also found in goats. Endemic in Great Britain and many other countries. Can be transmitted experimentally to other animals such as mice, the experimental model for work on spongiform encephalopathies.

SEs: Spongiform encephalopathies. Disorders affecting the brain in which small vacuoles or holes ('like a sponge') are apparent under the microscope.

SEAC: Spongiform Encephalopathy Advisory Committee (2nd Tyrrell Committee).

SEM: Standard error of the mean.

Sequence homology: The similarity or identity of nucleotide sequences, in genes of different individuals or species.

Sinc: The major gene that controls the incubation period of experimental scrapie in mice. Alleles s^7 and p^7.

Sip: Gene that controls the incubation period of natural and experimental scrapie in sheep. Alleles sA and pA.

SDS: Sodium dodecyl sulphate.

SSBP: Sheep scrapie brain pool.

STE: Stop-transfer effector.

Tau protein: A normal protein constituent of microtubules (cellular organelles) and found in excessive quantity in neurofibrillary tangles in the brain of patients with Alzheimer's disease and in the Indiana kindred of GSS patients.

TB: Tuberculosis.

Titre: The highest dilution of a material at which a biological effect can be detected, thus an approximate measure of concentration.

TME: Transmissible mink encephalopathy.

2D-NEPAGE/SDS-PAGE: Two dimensional gel electrophoresis, using, in the first dimension, *non-e*quilibrium pH gel electrophoresis and, in the second dimension, *s*odium *d*odecyl *s*ulphate polyacrylamide gel electrophoresis.

Transgenic: A technique in which all or parts of genes from one animal are inserted experimentally into the genes of the embryos of another. For example, mice can be given the *PrP* genes from hamsters.

Transmissible: Refers to agents or diseases that can be naturally or experimentally transmitted to the host species or other species.

TSE: Transmissible spongiform encephalopathy. Always fatal and thought to be caused by an unconventional infectious agent with a long incubation period. Not contagious except in sheep via the placenta, but can be experimentally transmitted to experimental animals. Some rare human forms are genetic (inherited) but are also transmissible.

Ubiquitin: A highly conserved protein found in normal cells which is synthesised in increasing amounts when cells are stressed and which functions as a co-factor for the degradation of abnormal or short-lived proteins. Ubiquitin is one of the heat shock proteins.

UK: United Kingdom.

US: United States (of America).

USDA: United States Department of Agriculture.

Vertical transmission: Transmission of disease from the male or female parent to offspring by genetic or environmental means.

VPC: Veterinary Products Committee.

Printed in the United Kingdom for HMSO
Dd 300148 C8 1/95